We would like to dedicate this book to:

Kevin, Chris, and Loryn

&

Elise, Justine, Ian, and George

And to the power of friends

We are thankful that our thirty plus year friendship has endured the completion of

this book and our other shared professional projects

"Too Busy to Diet", by Jacqueline King and Monica Joyce

@ 2013 by Jacqueline King and Monica Joyce

Library of Congress Control number: 2012918444
ISBN-13: 978-1480010581
ISBN-10: 1480010588

Acknowledgments

We'd like to thank the following dietetic students from University of Illinois at Chicago for reviewing and editing *Too Busy to Diet*: Lisa Taddei, Roxana Lorena Marcinas, and Terry Giordano.

Thank you also to Judy Joyce, sister and librarian who also helped review and edit.

Our gratitude to David Kromrey, MD: Resident at Resurrection Hospital, Chicago, Illinois for his careful review of the medical aspects of the book.

And to the following registered dietitians for their critiques, reviewing, and extra help:

Peggy Balboa, RD: Mariano's Fresh Market Dietitian

Maria Bournas, MS, RD: Mariano's Fresh Market Dietitian

Paulina Lowkis, RD, CDE

Julia Socke, RD, CDE: University of Chicago, Chicago, Illinois

Jamie Shish, RD, ATC/L

Thanks to Deb Funderwhite: photographer

Special thanks to Luz Chavez, Loyola University Dietetic Graduate student, for her patience and endless hours utilizing her computer graphics skills to create a book meeting our reader needs. We will be forever grateful.

Our special gratitude goes out to our thousands of patients and clients that we have provided nutrition counseling to over the years. Without them, there would be no *Too Busy to Diet*.

Thank You
Jackie and Monica

CONTENTS

INTRODUCTON

"SO MUCH TO DO, SO LITTLE TIME."

If those words sound familiar, then this book is for you: the busy professional, student, parent, volunteer, or retiree who packs a lot into a typical day. Never before has so much attention been focused on what we eat and how it impacts our health. The evidence is overwhelming that good nutrition and a sound exercise program can help you stay healthy and prevent disease. But how can we fit good nutrition and exercise into days that are already packed with demands and responsibilities?

Adding to the time crunch, the "typical" work day has also changed. Life's demands can begin before the crack of dawn and spill over into the evening hours. Technological advances enable us to work at any time of the day or night. In addition, work is often conducted during meals. Eating out becomes part of our busy lives, sometimes leaving us with little control over what, where, and when to eat.

However, what may appear to be an almost daunting task may actually be easier than you think. Combining a busy lifestyle with healthy eating and exercise can be a challenge but is not impossible. Some of the same skills you use to achieve balance in your typical day can be used to balance your health and nutrition. Planning and organizing are the key ingredients, so the most overwhelming tasks become easy and routine.

You asked. We've listened. Over the years we've listened carefully to you — our patients, family and friends. We know living healthy is a top priority. We've tried not to nag or preach, knowing the time pressures and that your daily lives and health are intrinsically intertwined. This patchwork of nutrition topics reflects your concerns.

A "back to basics" approach includes living healthy and concerns for planet earth. Research shows that our food choices can impact not only our health but the climate as well. Shifting your diet from meat and dairy to a vegetable-based one is healthy and can reduce carbon footprints. The 2010 Dietary Guidelines released on January 31, 2011 recommend that Americans reduce their salt, sugar and saturated fat. The guidelines encourage all Americans (ages 2 and older) to eat more fruits, vegetables, whole grains and low-fat dairy and seafood. The guidelines also emphasize reducing calories and increasing activity to promote a healthy weight.

This past decade we've been bombarded with nutrition research and information. We have tried to sift through the information so you can use *Too Busy to Diet* as a quick reference. You need not read this book cover to cover, or page by page. Instead, pick it up as needed. Throw it in the glove compartment of your car, briefcase, backpack, or diaper bag. Pull it out during lulls in your day to help you navigate through your busyness. It will help you stay motivated and focused on a healthy lifestyle. We recommend you turn to *"Too Busy to Diet"* as often as needed.

OUR WISH LIST FOR YOU

1. Cook healthy meals more often. Try a new recipe each week.

2. Eat more meals at home and sit down with the family (including your toddler).

3. Plan meals and snacks and shop for healthy foods at least once a week.

4. Discover simple, healthy recipes that you can make in less than 30 minutes.

5. Eat some of your favorite foods, some of the time: e.g., candy bar, ice cream.

6. Plant a garden or a pot with some favorite vegetables and herbs.

7. Don't spend money unnecessarily on supplements or trendy foods.

8. Avoid "junk nutrition"; look for reliable sources, e.g., registered dietitian.

9. Move more; take the stairs, walk around the office, clean the house.

10. Exercise daily at least 30 minutes.

11. Weigh yourself regularly.

Remember healthy eating is as easy as a quick trip to a local grocery store.

All you have to do is take some time out to plan a week of meals and snacks.

Shopping shouldn't take more than 15 to 20 minutes, and cooking a meal no more than 30 minutes.   No more "I'm too busy or too tired". You'll have more energy if you regularly exercise and you'll feel better if you are eating healthy.

Bon Appétit!

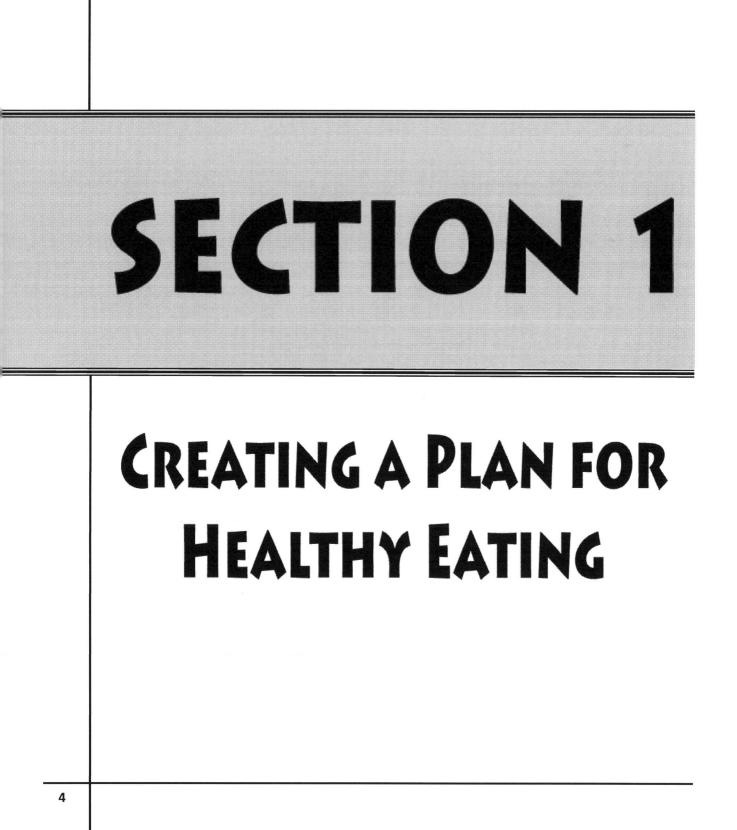

SECTION 1

CREATING A PLAN FOR HEALTHY EATING

HEALTHY EATING

"LET THE FOOD BE THE MEDICINE AND MEDICINE BE THE FOOD." -HIPPOCRATES

The connection between the foods we eat and our health was recognized as far back as Hippocrates. Now there has never been a time when we have been so encouraged to take charge of our health by eating healthy and exercising more. Our diets should be made up of a variety of foods, emphasizing fruits, vegetables, and whole grains. There is no mystery to weight loss and management. The key strategy for losing weight has never changed: decrease calorie intake and increase physical activity. Drive-thru, convenience foods, and take-out foods are all around. Preparing fresh, less processed foods at home is done less and less. Fast and easy recipes are available, but it takes planning and shopping. If planned correctly, healthy eating can save you time, calories, and money.

When interviewed, individuals who spent much of their time "on the run" identified the availability of nutritious meals and snacks as a top priority. They acknowledged that traveling and eating out can interfere with eating healthy and maintaining a healthy body weight. Eating on the go has led to an overweight epidemic we face today in America. We battle large portion sizes and calorie-dense foods that are easily accessible and often inexpensive; in most cases, we lose the battle and give in.

We are all moving less than ever. Many of us who have cars don't even think about walking to errands. Buses pick us up at the station and deposit us at our workplace, stealing the opportunity to walk. Some individuals complain of what's called "cubicilitis" or "computeritis", which in turn, limits our chances to move about during the workday. Down time is often spent at a computer or watching television. Too few of us meet the recommended 30 minutes or more of daily exercise. Because of this, every extra flight of stairs or 15 minutes of walking the family dog can really count.

CREATE A HEALTHY EATING PLAN

The path to healthy eating requires planning, shopping, and reading food labels to avoid eating whatever is in reach when in a rush. Choosing healthy foods requires a little effort. However, with practice, nutritious foods can quickly be incorporated into any lifestyle.

4 Steps to Creating a Healthy Meal Plan

1. **Plan:** Spend a few minutes once a week to map out a week's worth of dinner menus. Menus can be repeated. As you become more proficient at meal planning, try planning a month of menus to avoid repetition. See Menu Planning Chapter.

2. **Shop:** Create a weekly shopping list. Busy professionals often complain they don't have nutritious foods in the house. Plan and use a list. A trip to the grocery store will take less than 30 minutes. When writing a grocery list, add some low-calorie convenience snacks and meals as "back-ups." This will save time, money, and calories when you are too tired to prepare a meal. See Shopping Chapter.

3. **Read:** Read labels to avoid high calorie foods. Some convenience foods have large amounts of fat, sodium, and calories that can be easily avoided by reading the label. See Label Reading Chapter.

4. **Cook:** A simple yet nutritious meal can be prepared in less than thirty minutes. Cooking puts you in control of the quality and quantity of what you eat. Cooking can save calories and money, and often tastes better than prepared foods. Purchase a cookbook with quick and easy menu ideas and recipes, and get hooked on cooking. See Easy Dinners Chapter.

Deciding to eat healthy and to exercise regularly is done by choice rather than chance. The first step in embarking on a healthy lifestyle (or maintaining existing healthy lifestyle changes) is recognizing its importance. Make a commitment to incorporate healthy choices and make good health a priority. The *January 2011 AND Journal* reports that diets high in vegetables, fruits, whole grains, poultry, fish, and low-fat dairy foods may effect the quality of life and mortality in the older adult populations. This study showed that the adults following this type of diet had more healthy years of life. Once the decision is made, it is important to stay the course. Weight loss or weight maintenance is not a weeklong commitment; it is life-long. Consistency with a diet plan is crucial in order to obtain the desired results.

My Plate

MyPyramid, used for over 20 years, was recently replaced by the new icon, MyPlate. MyPlate was introduced to help Americans make easier food choices to ensure that they are achieving a healthy diet.

MyPlate can be found on the website: ChooseMyPlate.com. With the new website, the USDA emphasizes:

- Enjoying food but eating less
- Avoiding oversized portions
- Making half of your plate fruits and vegetables
- Drinking water instead of sugary drinks
- Switching to fat-free or low-fat milk
- Comparing the sodium content of foods
- Making half of your grains consumed whole grains
- Empty calories are now considered if you choose solid fats and added sugar.

MyPlate is a new tool to assist in making daily food choices based on recommended servings of the five different food groups. Registered dietitians welcome this change since most dietitians have been using the plate teaching tool for years. In both our practices, we are used to giving our patients the paper plate to formulate their food plan easily. The MyPlate continues to use the five food group approach because most Americans continue to fail to get adequate amounts of fiber, the vitamins A, C, and E, and the minerals calcium, magnesium, potassium in their daily diet. For this reason, MyPlate encourages a variety of foods, emphasizing a diet high in complex carbohydrates, low in sugar, and low in fats. Using MyPlate provides a diet adequate in vitamins and minerals. It also encourages a consumer to consider the portion of a serving when planning meals and snacks.

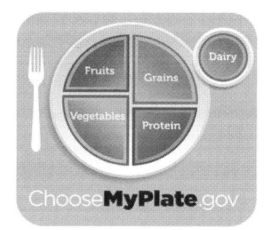

MyPlate is divided into five food groups, with each group represented by a different color.

5 Food Groups

1. Grains (orange): Make half your grains whole.
2. Vegetables (green): Vary your veggies.
3. Fruits (red): Focus on fruits.
4. Half of your plate should contain fruits and vegetables.
5. Dairy (blue): Get your calcium rich, low fat dairy choices.
6. Meat and Beans (purple): Go lean with protein.
7. Fats and Oils (yellow): Know the limits on fats, sugars, and salt.

In addition to a healthy diet, MyPlate also emphasizes the importance of physical activity. The incorporation of physical activity in every diet plan is extremely important in order to promote an overall healthy lifestyle.

MyPlate's recommendations are based on the sex, age, and level of activity for each individual person. Go to www.choosemyplate.com to figure out how many calories you need and how many portions of each food group you should be receiving. Under each food group, there is a reminder that if high fat items or sugar is added to the food choice, it is counted as empty calories from solid fats and added sugar. Refer to the chart on the next page for the amount of empty calories you should limit your diet to each day.

These new guidelines encourage individuals to maintain a desirable body weight. It highlights the importance of managing calories by focusing on portion control. MyPlate promotes weight loss by recommending that we lower our calories by eating less saturated fat and added sugars, as well as consuming less alcohol.

Managing weight, getting adequate nutrition, and participating in a regular exercise program are all part of being healthy.

Estimated calories for those who are not physically active		
Age and gender	Total daily calorie needs*	Daily limit for empty calories
Children 2-3 yrs	1000 cals	135**
Children 4-8 yrs	1200-1400 cals	120
Girls 9-13 yrs	1600 cals	120
Boys 9-13 yrs	1800 cals	160
Girls 14-18 yrs	1800 cals	160
Boys 14-18 yrs	2200 cals	265
Females 19-30 yrs	2000 cals	260
Males 19-30 yrs	2400 cals	330
Females 31-50 yrs	1800 cals	160
Males 31-50 yrs	2200 cals	265
Females 51+ yrs	1600 cals	120
Males 51+ yrs	2000 cals	260

* These amounts are appropriate for individuals who get less than 30 minutes of moderate physical activity most days. Those who are more active need more total calories, and have a higher limit for empty calories. To find your personal total calorie needs and empty calories limit, enter your information into "My Daily Food Plan."

** The limit for empty calories is higher for children 2 and 3 years old than it is for some older children, because younger children have lower nutrient needs and smaller recommended intakes from the basic food groups.

VEGETARIAN: TO BE OR NOT TO BE

"NOTHING WILL BENEFIT HUMAN HEALTH AND INCREASE CHANCES FOR SURVIVAL OF LIFE ON EARTH AS MUCH AS THE EVOLUTION TO A VEGETARIAN DIET." -ALBERT EINSTEIN

Vegetarian Diet Questions: Test your knowledge by answering <u>True</u> or <u>False</u> to the following questions:

1. I am not a vegetarian if I eat eggs or dairy products on a daily basis.

2. As a vegetarian, I will never be able to get adequate amounts of vitamin B-12 from my diet.

3. I do not have to worry about getting enough iron in my diet because I eat a lot of high iron-containing vegetables.

4. If I combine foods such as rice and beans or dairy and bread, I will be able to get complete protein in my diet.

Thinking about becoming a vegetarian? People choose to be a vegetarian for different reasons, including:

- Don't enjoy eating meat
- Animal welfare or environmental concerns
- General concern about health
- Belief that a diet high in complex carbohydrates and fiber is healthier than one high in animal protein and saturated fat
- Religious beliefs

Concerned about the planet earth? Vegetarians often consider animal processing, types of feeds provided (kind of like a hot dog...Don't tell me what's in it), and the carbon emissions produced by cows and livestock to be a major concern. Vegetarian Science Daily (April 21, 2008) reports that Carnegie Mellon researchers report that shifting from the American diet to a vegetable-based diet would reduce greenhouse gas emissions equivalent to driving 8,000 miles per year. Whatever the reason, when eating in a vegetarian style, it is important to focus on variety of foods for a nutritionally sound diet.

A vegetarian diet consists primarily of whole grains, fruits, vegetables, legumes, and meat substitutes. There are different types of vegetarians. Some people who choose to be vegetarians do not eat any meat or animal products, including fowl or seafood, or any products containing these foods. Others do eat dairy products, eggs, and fish. If you are a vegetarian that limits or eliminates animal choices, be sure to include a variety of foods to ensure you are receiving the right vitamins and minerals. Plant sources that include legumes such as chick peas, beans and soy can help provide a healthy diet.

A 2009 position statement by the Academy of Nutrition and Dietetics states that appropriately planned vegetarian diets, including total vegetarian or vegan diets, are healthful, nutritionally adequate, and may provide health benefits in the prevention and treatment of certain diseases. Well-planned vegetarian diets are appropriate for individuals during all stages of the lifecycle, including pregnancy, lactation, infancy, childhood, and adolescence, and for athletes.

WHICH "VEGETARIAN" ARE YOU?

Eating vegetarian can mean many different things. Making the decision to become a vegetarian is the first step in a different way of eating and is just one part of the equation. Next, you'll need to determine which type of vegetarian diet you want to follow. You should have an understanding of the eating patterns that make up all the vegetarian diets. Some vegetarians include different types of animal foods.

Lacto-Ovo Vegetarian	Most popular and is the easiest to follow Includes cheese, eggs, milk, and grains
Lacto-Vegetarians	Includes cheese, milk, and yogurt Eliminates eggs and foods that contain eggs
Vegan	Eliminates eggs and dairy products, as well as foods that contain protein derivatives such as whey and casein Avoids honey since it comes from bees Vegans may need to take a daily B-12 supplement since animal foods are the main source of this vitamin (more on this below)
Semi-Vegetarian (aka: Flexitarian)	Picks and chooses different parts of a vegetarian diet Plant-based with the occasional use of fish, poultry, or meats
Zen-Macrobiotic	Limited to a variety of grains and very little fluid Not nutritionally adequate
Macrobiotic	Grains, legumes, nuts, and some vegetables are used Soy products and Asian condiments are used frequently Fish may be included by some individuals Avoids dairy, eggs, and some vegetables

BENEFITS AND CONCERNS OF VEGETARIAN EATING

Benefits: Including health and weight management benefits

1. Vegetarians typically maintain a desirable body weight and have a lower body mass index.

2. Vegetarians also typically have less cardiovascular disease, cancers, and gastrointestinal disorders.

3. Vegetarians have lower blood pressure, low-density lipoprotein cholesterol levels and lower rates of hypertension and Type 2 Diabetes.

4. Vegetarian diets tend to be higher in fiber, magnesium, potassium, Vitamins C and E, folate, carotenoids, flavonoids and other phytochemicals.

5. Vegetarian diets tend to be lower in saturated fat and cholesterol.

Nutritional Concerns:

Deficiencies can be avoided by choosing a wide variety of foods. The vitamins and minerals noted are found in meats and can also be found in plant sources. Make sure your diet contains complete protein sources by combining whole grain breads, rice, and legumes.

Deficiencies Possible:

- ✓ B Vitamins
- ✓ Iron
- ✓ Protein
- ✓ Calcium
- ✓ Vitamin D
- ✓ Zinc
- ✓ Iodine
- ✓ Omega-3 Fatty Acids

Vitamin B-12

Purpose: necessary for red blood cell maturation, nerve function, and DNA synthesis.

Deficiency Symptoms: anemia, dizziness, paleness, fatigue, neuropathy (nerve damage), and in more severe instances mental impairment, dementia, and paranoia.

Sources:

✓ Lacto-ovo-vegetarians obtain B-12 from dairy foods and eggs. Vegans must obtain B-12 from regular use of B-12 fortified foods and B-12 supplements.

✓ Fortified soy and rice beverages, some meat analogs and breakfast cereals or Red Star Vegetarian Support Formula nutritional yeast provide B-12.

✓ Good sources are milk, eggs, and cheese. Since these are animal products, vegans and those following macrobiotic diets will need to get this vitamin from B-12 enriched cereals and fortified soy products like vegetarian patties or by taking a vitamin supplement.

✓ Multivitamin

Iron

Purpose: Provides oxygen binding in red blood cells to be carried to the body. Absorption of iron from plants is affected by inhibitors and enhancers.

Inhibits Absorption: Calcium, fiber, phytates found in raw soy and lima beans, polyphenols found in tea, coffee, herbs teas and cocoa.

Enhances Absorption: Vitamin C and organic acids found in fruits and vegetables.

Deficiency Symptoms: Some of the same symptoms as B12 deficiency, anemia, dizziness, paleness, and fatigue. Very common deficiency in women.

Recommended Intake: For vegetarians, recommended intake is 1.8 times that of non-vegetarians because of the lower availability of iron in non-animal products.

Sources:

✓ Enriched whole-grain products like cereals and breads, dried peas, beans, and lentils.

✓ Look for kidney beans, black-eyed peas, and turnip greens.

✓ Leafy green vegetables and some dried fruits (raisins, apricots, prunes), and eggs have iron.

Protein

Purpose: Protein in the diet helps make up the structure and function of our body, from our DNA, cells, nerves, our skin, muscles, hair, etc.

Deficiency Symptoms: Decreased pigmentation of hair, hair can easily fall out (pluckable). Since B vitamins are part of most protein products, anemia may accompany.

Recommended Intake: A vegetarian diet that includes eggs and dairy products will usually provide enough protein in the diet. When avoiding meat, it is important to consume foods containing complete proteins. Combining legumes with a variety of grains can provide those complete proteins.

Sources:

✓ Milk, eggs, nuts, and beans are sources of protein. By eating a variety of plant proteins over the course of a day, all the essential amino acids can be provided.

✓ Soy is the best known of the plant proteins. It contains all of the essential amino acids, making it a complete protein. In fact, soy is the only food with plant protein that is equal in quality to the protein found in meat and eggs.

✓ Tempeh is a soy protein that also provides fiber, B vitamins, and iron. Its mild flavor makes it compatible with many dishes such as casseroles, stir-fries and chili.

✓ Soy yogurt is a portable soy product that can make a great snack and is high in nutrition.

✓ Tofu or bean curd is a good source of protein and calcium. It most often is an ingredient in "meat analogs" also known as meat substitutes and veggie burgers. Be sure to read labels to find out.

Calcium

Purpose: Dietary intake is needed for increased bone mass and density during puberty and to maintain bone health in adults. Calcium is also required for nerve transmission and regulation in function of muscles, especially those of the heart.

Deficiency Symptoms: Low dietary intakes may contribute to decreased bone mass. If the diet is low in both vitamin D and calcium, it can contribute to osteomalacia. Vegetarians tend to have high intakes of calcium often higher than those of non-vegetarians. Vegans tend to have lower calcium intakes with a 30% higher risk for bone fracture.

Sources:

✓ Soy milk, rice milk and breakfast cereals.

✓ Dairy products are the best source of calcium.

✓ Dark green leafy vegetables, such as spinach, collard greens, turnips, kale, bok choy, Chinese cabbage, and broccoli.

✓ Tofu enriched with calcium.

Vitamin D

Purpose: Important role in the maintenance of calcium levels, contributing to healthy bones and teeth. Also, more than 50 genes are known to be regulated by vitamin D.

Deficiency Symptoms: Rickets in children and osteomalacia in adults. Calcitriol is the active form of vitamin D in the body. Our bodies convert cholesterol in the skin into vitamin D using the sun's ultra-violet light. People living in northern climates, individuals with dark skin, and those who use large amounts of sunscreen could be deficient in vitamin D. Also, vegan and macrobiotic diets that do not include fortified foods or supplements may not supply enough vitamin D.

Sources:

✓ The Sun

✓ Vitamin D-fortified milk and orange juice, soy or rice drinks, cereal, margarines and many soy products.

✓ Herring, Sardines, Salmon, Shrimp

✓ If exposure to sunlight is limited use a supplement of Vitamin D.

Zinc

Purpose: Zinc is an essential trace mineral important in growth and development, immune response, neurological function and reproduction.

Deficiency Symptoms: Strict vegetarians may need zinc supplementation because plant staples are a majority of their diet. Phytic acid, found in plants and other whole grain products, reduce zinc absorption. If yeast is used to leaven whole grain bread, zinc becomes available for absorption by the body. Mild deficiency can cause impaired physical and neuropsychological development and inability to fight infection, especially in children.

Sources:

✓ Leavened whole grain bread products

✓ Shellfish

✓ Nuts and legumes

✓ Eggs and dairy, cheese, soy products

✓ Beans (white, kidney, chick peas)

✓ Pumpkin seeds

Iodine

Purpose: Essential trace mineral concentrated in the thyroid gland for synthesizing several thyroid hormones.

Deficiency Symptoms: Goiter, which is a large visible lump on the neck, caused by the increase in Thyroid-Stimulating Hormone (TSH). This is also a symptom of iodine excess. See your physician if this situation exists. Plant- based diets can be low in iodine. Since some vegans may not use iodized salt or sea vegetables, they may be at risk for iodine deficiency.

Sources:

✓ Depends upon the soil where food is grown. Mountainous areas and river deltas are usually deficient in iodine.

✓ Sea food and seaweed

✓ Milk

✓ Iodized salt (not present in sea salt)

Omega-3 Fatty Acids

Purpose: Fatty acids eicosapentanoic acid (EPA) and docosahexaenoic acid (DHA) are omega-3 (n-3) fatty acids and are known for their important role in cardiovascular health and eye and brain development.

Deficiency Symptoms: Vegans tend to have lower levels of EPA and DHA. Vegetarian diets are usually high in omega-6 fatty acids but may be low in n-3 fatty acids.

Sources of Omega-3 Fatty Acids:

✓   DHA Fortified soymilk and breakfast bars

✓   Fatty fish, such as tuna, salmon, mackerel, sardines

✓   Fish oil supplements

✓   Walnuts

VEGETARIANS ON THE MOVE!

Following a vegetarian diet is easier than ever. Product availability has grown with demand and consumption of processed vegetarian foods such as meat analogs, nondairy milks and vegetarian entrees. More and more fortified foods, including breakfast cereals, juices, and soy milk, are appearing on grocery store shelves. Grocery stores and natural food stores are making it easier than ever to get the right nutrients.

Fortified food choices make it easier to get the right nutrients.

Tips for the Vegetarian on the Go

Don't let a hectic schedule or frequent traveling prevent you from adopting a vegetarian eating style. It is much easier to follow a vegetarian diet than it once was.

Foods Offered. The variety of foods offered at grocery stores is greater than ever. The frozen food section even offers vegan meals. Look for whole grains and avoid high sodium meals. Two reliable brands are Amy's and Dr. Praeger's. Use canned soybeans as you would other beans.

Quick Meals. Boxed mixes, such as rice pilaf, risotto, and vegetable chili, can turn into a healthy vegan meal in no time at all. Again, check labels to avoid the highly processed mixes. Add a vegetable, a salad, and fruit to make it complete.

Fast Foods. Many fast food restaurants have meatless alternatives that can fit easily into a vegetarian diet. For instance, Wendy's serves baked potatoes with cheese and broccoli. Other meatless meals on the run are cheese pizza with a salad, or a bean burrito. Be aware of sodium and fat when choosing from fast food restaurants. Try to balance the day with low-fat, low-sodium foods.

Restaurants. No need to avoid restaurant dining. Plan ahead to find restaurants that have a variety of meatless menu items. Many offer vegetarian menu alternatives. If a restaurant does not offer vegetarian items, you can often create a meal by asking if the chef could eliminate meat fillings or toppings. Or, try choosing a variety of meatless appetizers or side dishes.

Try ethnic foods. Some ethnic dishes (especially Italian, Mexican, and Chinese) can be easily incorporated into a vegetarian eating style. Vegetable lasagna, cheese ravioli, and manicotti stuffed with spinach and cheese are vegetarian Italian meals. Bean tacos or burritos, cheese quesadillas, and vegetable fajitas are popular meatless Mexican foods. Asian and Indian restaurants offer a variety of vegetable dishes as well.

Quantity service, travel and banquets. When traveling by air or attending a banquet, vegetarian meals can be reserved in advance. With the large number of vegetarians, most banquets set aside vegetarian dishes "just in case." International flights, or flights still offering meal service, also offer vegetarian meals which can be requested when reserving your ticket.

Car Travel. If you are traveling by car, a roadside restaurant known best for a meat and potatoes type of menu will most likely also have items such as grilled cheese sandwiches, peanut butter and jelly sandwiches, macaroni and cheese, salads, meatless soups, or baked potatoes that can make a quick meal. Other meal options include bean or vegetable soup with a salad and a roll, or a cottage cheese and fruit platter. Snack on roasted soy nuts or add soy nuts to a trail mix.

Tips to Help You Be Successful

Here are some tips to ensure success in vegetarian cooking, eating, and keeping the right foods on hand

Begin by decreasing meat dishes

For beginner vegetarians, try increasing complex carbohydrates, like whole-wheat rice and pasta, and decreasing the amount of meat you are eating. Try replacing one meal per day with a meatless meal. For example, try cheese ravioli with marinara sauce, a salad, and bread or a hearty bean soup with a roll and salad.

Provide Variety and Balance

Variety is the key. Avoid eating the same foods over and over. Choose a variety of fruits and vegetables and low fat dairy products. Replace whole grain flour with soy. Make burgers out of tofu, beans, and brown rice.

Vegetarian Recipes and Cookbooks

There are many websites that provide vegetarian recipes. Purchase a vegetarian cookbook and select a handful of recipes you enjoy and that are easy to prepare. Practice fixing different foods and have a friend over to try them out.

Quick Veggie Dishes

Vegetarian cooking can be quick and easy if you plan ahead. If you haven't much time, prepare some pasta which cooks up in minutes. Add a pesto sauce or sauté fresh tomatoes with onion and garlic for a quick sauce. Add parmesan cheese and a salad. Try tofu in a stir fry. Add soybeans or tofu to chili or casserole.

Back Up Foods

Have back-up foods in the freezer for when you are too tired or busy to cook. A frozen meatless meal can be quick, healthy, and low in calories. Stock your freezer with cheese ravioli, tortellini, and gnocchi. Add a salad, bread, and vegetables for a complete meal.

Soups

Keep a variety of meatless canned soups on hand. Many soups contain both legumes and vegetables. But watch the sodium content.

Snacks

Find meatless snacks to grab when you get hungry. Some nutritious options include nuts (especially almonds, walnuts, and soy nuts), fruit, yogurt, granola bars, and pretzels. Make your own trail mix from soy nuts, raisins, almonds, and apricots.

*Soy snack ideas from The Soy Connection Spring 2011

Nutrition Tips:

*Choose mostly whole grains.
*Eat a variety of foods from each of the food groups.
*Adults age 70 and younger need 600 IU of vitamin D daily.
  Sources include fortified foods (such as some soymilks) or a vitamin D supplement.
*Sources of iodine include iodized salt (3/8 teaspoon daily) or
  an iodine supplement (150 micrograms).
*See www.vrg.org for recipes and more details.

Vegan
MY ^PLATE

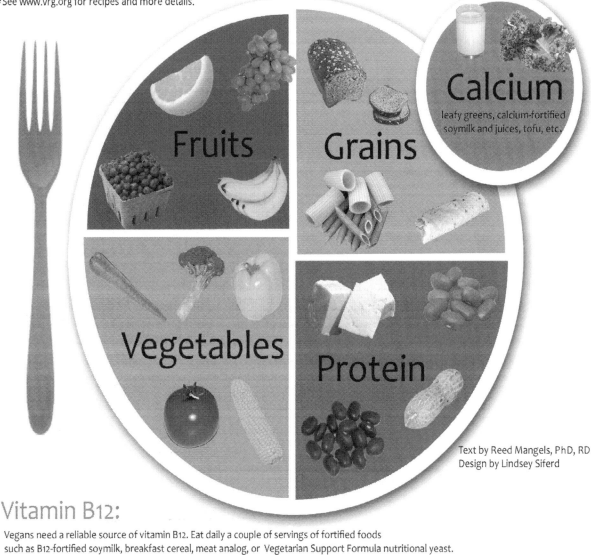

Text by Reed Mangels, PhD, RD
Design by Lindsey Siferd

Vitamin B12:

Vegans need a reliable source of vitamin B12. Eat daily a couple of servings of fortified foods
such as B12-fortified soymilk, breakfast cereal, meat analog, or Vegetarian Support Formula nutritional yeast.
Check the label for fortification. If fortified foods are not eaten daily,
you should take a vitamin B12 supplement (25 micrograms daily).

Note:

Like any food plan, this should only serve as a general guide for adults.
The plan can be modified according to your own personal needs. This is not personal
medical advice. Individuals with special health needs should consult a registered
dietitian or a medical doctor knowledgeable about vegan nutrition.

VRg. The Vegetarian
Resource Group P.O. Box 1463 Baltimore, MD 21203 www.vrg.org (410) 366-8343

Table 2: Protein Content of Selected Vegan Foods

FOOD	AMOUNT	PROTEIN(gm)	PROTEIN(gm/100 cal)
Tempeh	1 cup	41	9.3
Seitan	3 ounces	31	22.1
Soybeans, cooked	1 cup	29	9.6
Lentils, cooked	1 cup	18	7.8
Black beans, cooked	1 cup	15	6.7
Kidney beans, cooked	1 cup	13	6.4
Veggie burger	1 patty	13	13.0
Chickpeas, cooked	1 cup	12	4.2
Veggie baked beans	1 cup	12	5.0
Pinto beans, cooked	1 cup	12	5.7
Black-eyed peas, cooked	1 cup	11	6.2
Tofu, firm	4 ounces	11	11.7
Lima beans, cooked	1 cup	10	5.7
Quinoa, cooked	1 cup	9	3.5
Tofu, regular	4 ounces	9	10.6
Bagel	1 med. (3 oz)	9	3.9
Peas, cooked	1 cup	9	6.4
Textured Vegetable Protein (TVP), cooked	1/2 cup	8	8.4
Peanut butter	2 Tbsp	8	4.3
Veggie dog	1 link	8	13.3
Spaghetti, cooked	1 cup	8	3.7
Almonds	1/4 cup	8	3.7
Soy milk, commercial, plain	1 cup	7	7.0
Soy yogurt, plain	6 ounces	6	4.0
Bulgur, cooked	1 cup	6	3.7
Sunflower seeds	1/4 cup	6	3.3
Whole wheat bread	2 slices	5	3.9
Cashews	1/4 cup	5	2.7
Almond butter	2 Tbsp	5	2.4
Brown rice, cooked	1 cup	5	2.1
Spinach, cooked	1 cup	5	13.0
Broccoli, cooked	1 cup	4	6.8
Potato	1 med. (6 oz)	4	2.7

Sources: USDA Nutrient Database for Standard Reference, Release 18, 2005 and manufacturers' information.

The recommendation for protein for adult males vegans is around 56-70 grams per day; for adult female vegans it is around 46-58 grams per day (see text).

Answers to Vegetarian Questions

1. False. A lacto-ovo vegetarian diet includes eggs and dairy.

2. False. Although more difficult, it is possible to obtain adequate amounts of B-12 if you eat vegetarian sources of B-12 or take a supplement.

3. False. It is difficult to get enough iron through vegetables since they are not a good source of iron, and the iron is not absorbed as well. Therefore, iron fortified cereals, other iron fortified foods, or supplements should be consumed.

4. True.

MEDITERRANEAN DIET

"You Don't Have to Cook Fancy or Complicated Masterpieces - Just Good Food from Fresh Ingredients." - Julia Child

Perhaps the love affair with food that Mediterranean people hold has led to this naturally heart-healthy way of eating. Despite the diversity of this region, the people have embraced a similar eating pattern that is not only healthy, but tastes great. This diet includes an abundance of plant foods including vegetables, fruits, legumes, whole grains, and nuts. It also contains several sources of omega-3 fatty acids such as fatty fish, greens such as kale and spinach, and walnuts which help protect against heart disease. Olive oil, which is also a main staple of the diet, is a rich source of omega-6 fatty acids. The diet is rich in vitamins, minerals, antioxidants, polyphenols, and fiber.

Studies from the last few decades have shown that despite a moderate to high intake of salt, fat, and alcohol (red wine), the people of this region have a much lower rate of cardiovascular disease than people in the United States. The Lyon Heart Study showed that there was a 70% lower incidence of nonfatal repeat heart attacks in the group that followed a Mediterranean diet versus the group using a low-fat diet that was high in polyunsaturated fat. A study in the New England Journal of Medicine in 2008 demonstrated a greater weight loss in those individuals who followed a Mediterranean diet. Another study in The British Medical Journal in the same year showed a reduced risk of dying from cancer and cardiovascular disease, as well as less risk for Parkinson's and Alzheimer's diseases.

Fruits, Vegetables, and Whole Grains: These items make up the main meal. Some meals are completely meatless. Sauces are often made with yogurt, fresh vegetables, and herbs. Fruit can end a meal as a dessert and be used as a between meal snack.

Oils, Fats, and Meats: Total fat in the diet is 25% to 35% of calories. Saturated fat is approximately 8% or less of total calories. Over half the fat in the diet is from monounsaturated fat, the *good* fat. Olive orchards make up the landscape of some of these regions making olive oil the oil of choice. Examples of these fats are:

- Extra-virgin and virgin olive oils are the least processed oils, so they contain the highest amounts of polyphenols and antioxidants.

- Red meats are not used as frequently as fish and poultry, lowering the overall intake of saturated fat and cholesterol.

- Fish is eaten two to three times per week. Good choices are tuna, salmon, mackerel, herring, and trout due to their higher content of omega-3 fatty acids.

Portions: As we've said all along, it's not just choosing healthy foods, but also managing portions. When visiting any of these countries, one is often surprised at the smaller portion sizes. Snacking is rare and coffee or espresso breaks are usually not accompanied by a dessert or snack.

Seasoning: Fresh herbs and spices are used to season foods, rather than salt.

Natural Foods: Processed foods and fast food are not a part of everyday life in these countries.

Wine: Moderate intake of wine is enjoyed with meals.

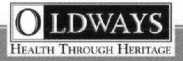

Mediterranean Diet Pyramid

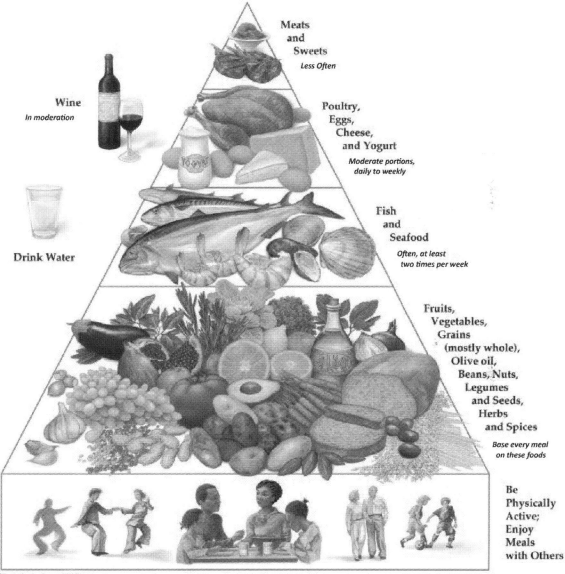

Meats
and
Sweets
Less Often

Wine
In moderation

Poultry,
Eggs,
Cheese,
and Yogurt
*Moderate portions,
daily to weekly*

Drink Water

Fish
and
Seafood
*Often, at least
two times per week*

Fruits,
Vegetables,
Grains
(mostly whole),
Olive oil,
Beans, Nuts,
Legumes
and Seeds,
Herbs
and Spices
*Base every meal
on these foods*

Be
Physically
Active;
Enjoy
Meals
with Others

Illustration by George Middleton

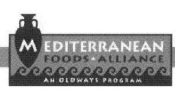

What Makes this a Good Diet?

High in complex carbohydrates, making it naturally high in fiber, low in fat, and rich in many different nutrients. Complex carbohydrates come from:

- Fruits and vegetables.

- Breads, pastas, rice, whole grains (such as quinoa and couscous), and cereals.

- Beans, nuts, and seeds.

Low in saturated fat:

- Fish, poultry, and dairy are the main sources of protein and are used sparingly.

- There is a low consumption of red meat.

- Saturated and Trans-Fats have been shown to increase cholesterol levels and contribute to heart disease.

High in monounsaturated fat from olive oil, olives, and canola oil:

- High in omega-3 fatty acids.

- Olive oil has beneficial anti-inflammatory properties.

- Monounsaturated fat has been shown to reduce LDL cholesterol levels.

High in omega-3 fatty acids:

- Sources include fish, olive oil, and nuts (especially walnuts).

- Omega-3 fatty acids have been shown to lower triglycerides, improving blood vessel health.

Moderate intake of wine:

- Red wine has been shown to increase HDL (good) cholesterol.

- Good source of the phytochemical *resveratrol*, which has been shown to prevent clotting and plaque formation in arteries.

- Limit to 5 ounces per day for women and 10 ounces per day for men.

Most diets come and go quickly because they have no roots or science to back them. Yet the Mediterranean diet and the lifestyle that accompanies it has been linked to good health for ages.

How Can I Adopt this Diet?

1. Try easy-to-prepare fish and poultry recipes. Baking, broiling, and grilling are fast and require little preparation. Cooking yourself can take less time than eating a meal out.

2. Find a handful of easy to prepare recipes that reflect this eating style. For some easy, delicious recipes, try Alexander Lindberg, MD, *Eating the Greek Way* or *The Mediterranean diabetes Cookbook: A flavorful, Low-Fat, Heart Healthy Approach to Cooking.*

3. Cut back red meat servings to 3 servings per week.

4. Use herbs and spices to enhance flavor and you'll use less salt.

5. Make pasta dishes for a fast and easy meal. A meatless sauce can be prepared in minutes by sautéing fresh tomatoes, onions, and other vegetables in olive oil. Use seasonal vegetables in your sauce to vary your recipe and keep meals seeming fresh and new.

6. Use olive oil when cooking and on salads.

7. Cook fresh or frozen vegetables for a side dish.

8. Finish off your meal with some fresh fruit and low-fat cheese.

9. Try a handful of walnuts or almonds as a snack or sprinkle on a dish.

10. Check with your doctor about adding a glass of red wine with a meal.

VITAMINS & MINERALS

"ADAM AND EVE ATE THE FIRST VITAMINS, INCLUDING THE PACKAGE". - E.R.SQUIBB

Vitamin/Mineral Supplement Questions: Test your knowledge by answering <u>True</u> or <u>False</u> to the following questions:

1. It is important to take daily vitamin supplements because they can boost your energy.

2. A vitamin supplement is probably not necessary if you are eating a variety of foods.

3. Taking vitamins can substitute for eating a healthy diet.

4. Vitamins can be important for those with some disease processes, a poor appetite, during pregnancy, and if following a strict vegetarian diet.

5. Doubling your daily vitamin intake will make you healthier.

6. Taking single vitamin and mineral supplements is better than taking a multivitamin supplement.

7. Natural vitamins are superior to synthetic vitamins.

VITAMIN AND MINERAL SUPPLEMENTS

Dietary supplements are big business in America. In fact, in 2007, as reported in Nutrition Business Journal, Americans spent $4.5 billion on multivitamins. Vitamins and minerals are essential to life and a healthy lifestyle. As a general rule, it is always recommended to obtain the vitamins and minerals needed every day from a diet containing a variety of healthy foods. However, it is important to be aware of the possible need to supplement your diet in order to prevent deficiencies. No matter if the vitamins and minerals come from the food you eat or a supplement, meeting the RDA each day should be your number one priority. Most dietitians would agree that consuming a well-balanced diet is the best guarantee for obtaining optimal levels of vitamins and minerals. They encourage this due to research that shows that a daily multivitamin may be a big waste of money. Research from the Women's Health Initiative has found that vitamin consumers are no healthier than those who did not consume vitamins in the development of cancer, heart disease, and stroke. This study involved over 160,000 mid-life women. The research also found that women with poor diets were not helped with the use of multivitamins in preventing cancer, heart disease, or stroke. Some health professionals may recommend vitamin/mineral use for individuals at increased risk of developing nutrient deficiencies including those who are pregnant, lactating, dieting, peri-menopausal women, elderly, and those with chronic diseases. They also might recommend their use by individuals who are at increased risk of developing nutritional deficiencies due to the following:

- Abusing alcohol, drugs, tobacco

- Using long-term medications

- Experiencing stress

- Consuming less than 2000 calories / day

- Skipping meals

- Making poor food choices

The recent research is not as encouraging regarding their use. It is important to remember that vitamin/mineral supplement use was started in the early 1900's. This was due to the fact that it was difficult to obtain a wide assortment of fruits and vegetables year round. It is highly unlikely for anyone to be seriously deficient today due to the number of packaged foods that are vitamin and mineral enriched.

Vitamin-mineral preparations are called dietary supplements. They are designed to be added to a normal diet to allow an increase in the total daily intake of one or more vitamins and minerals. Vitamin-mineral supplements might be helpful in boosting nutrient intake to ensure optimal health. Many individuals have concerns about their need for vitamin-mineral supplements because with so many options, it can be difficult to know what the right supplement is for their needs. Beware of individuals selling supplements. Keep in mind that their motivation is often their own financial gain, not your health. Registered dietitians are the best source of information; they can evaluate your diet and let you know if there are any deficiencies that need to be corrected by either diet or supplements. They can also give you ideas for foods that you can eat to boost your vitamin/mineral intake.

VITAMINS

Vitamins can be classified into two categories, both of which are essential to living. They are water-soluble and fat-soluble vitamins. Water-soluble vitamins usually help regulate metabolism, produce and release energy, make red blood cells, strengthen the immune system, and serve as antioxidants. Fat-soluble vitamins are necessary to ensure proper cell growth, healthy vision, strong bone development, and antioxidant protection. Coenzymes, such as the water-soluble vitamins (except Vitamin C), are factors that help enzymes function in the body. Antioxidants are substances that protect cells from damage done by free radicals within the body.

There are nine water-soluble vitamins needed in the body. These vitamins are found in the watery portions of foods, are lost easily when food is overcooked, and do

Water-Soluble Vitamins
• Vitamin C
• the B Vitamins:
• thiamin (B1)
• riboflavin (B2)
• niacin (B3)
• pantothenic acid (B5)
• pyridoxine (B6)
• biotin (B7)
• folic acid (B9)
• cyanocobalamin (B12)

not require fat to be absorbed. Water-soluble vitamins mix easily in the blood and are excreted in the urine with excess use. So only small amounts are stored in the body. Therefore, it is important to note that water soluble vitamins must be continually supplied in the diet on a daily basis to avoid deficiencies.

The fat-soluble vitamins are A, D, E, and K, and are absorbed with fat from our food. They can accumulate in toxic amounts in your body because they are not excreted in urine like water-soluble vitamins. Vitamin K can actually be toxic in individuals on anticoagulant medications when taken in large amounts long-term. Vitamins A and D have also been shown to be toxic with doses 15 and 5 times the RDA, respectively. Recent research is showing that one vitamin that should not be missed is Vitamin D. Chapter 13 has more information about this vitamin. It is of particular concern in areas with low exposure to sunshine. It is being praised due to research showing a reduction in heart attacks, a reduction in at least a dozen types of cancer, and improved absorption of calcium. Large doses of vitamin E have not been found to be toxic. However, taking amounts greater than 800 I.U. per day have not been found to be beneficial.

Megavitamin therapy is the use of supplements in amounts that exceed the recommended daily allowance (RDA) by 10 times or more. This practice began when individuals adopted the misconception that if a small amount of a nutrient is good, a large amount would be even better. Megavitamin therapy is generally unnecessary and can be expensive. The biggest risk is that it can be harmful to the body, especially with the accumulation of fat-soluble vitamins.

MINERALS

Minerals, like vitamins, are also essential to life. The roles of minerals in the body are similar to vitamins, including serving as cofactors, releasing and making energy, acting as antioxidants, and regulating metabolism. However, there are other functions, such as acid-base balance, muscle contraction, and nerve conduction, which are mainly controlled by minerals, not vitamins. The amount of mineral absorbed by the body is largely dependent on the "bioavailability" of that mineral. In other words, different factors such as the other nutrients eaten along with the mineral, the form of the mineral, and whether the mineral is chemically bound to something else could affect how much mineral your body absorbs.

Just like some vitamins, large doses of certain minerals, even as little as a few times the RDA can be dangerous if they accumulate in your tissues. They can actually cause a secondary deficiency of other minerals. For example, iron taken in large amounts can cause constipation, stomach and gastrointestinal upset, and can accumulate in the liver, pancreas, and other organs, causing a condition called hemosiderosis. Large amounts of selenium can cause nervous system disorders, liver problems, or kidney disorders. Large doses of zinc can cause a copper deficiency because the two minerals compete for absorption in the small intestine.

Individuals should not consume more than three times the RDA from vitamin –mineral supplements. Taking doses that are anywhere from 10 to 1,000 times the RDA for long periods of time can have detrimental health effects. With the exception of iron, minerals are generally better absorbed with meals. Iron, however; is absorbed much better on an empty stomach.

Mega-dose Dangers

- **Excessive Vitamin A or niacin intake can cause liver damage.**

- **Excessive vitamin C or zinc intake can reduce the immune response and encourage kidney stone formation.**

- **Excessive vitamin B6 intake can cause irreversible nerve damage.**

- **Excessive pantothenic acid can cause diarrhea.**

Beware of the product Vitaminwater by the Coca Cola Company. This product touts improving health and providing a healthy state of physical and mental well being. Vitaminwater has over 33 grams of sugar and 132 calories in a 20 ounce bottle. Vitaminwater names only two of its main ingredients: vitamins and water. It omits its significant ingredient, sugar that contributes a significant amount of calories to the daily diet, especially if multiple bottles are consumed each day.

- **Buffered vitamins** - Some vitamins (in particular, vitamin C) are acidic and can irritate the digestive tract if taken in mega-doses. Buffered vitamins have a compound added to neutralize the acid and make them less irritating.

- **Chelated minerals** - These minerals are attached to another substance to enhance absorption in the body. However, the acidic stomach environment usually breaks this attachment, so chelation generally does not improve absorption. There are a few cases, however, where chelation does enhance the mineral's effectiveness. The chelated forms of iron fumerate and zinc gluconate have been found to be less irritating to the stomach and intestine than other chelated minerals. This reduces stomach upsets and constipation when taken in large amounts. The chelated form of chromium (chromium picolinate) is also very well absorbed.

- **Chewable vitamins** - Chewable vitamins are an easy way to encourage children (who may not yet be able to swallow pills) to take a daily multivitamin. However, since children's multivitamins taste like candy, their vitamin consumption should be carefully monitored. A child's smaller size can increase susceptibility to vitamin toxicity. Be aware that the exposure of the tooth enamel to vitamin C in chewable vitamins can wear away enamel and increase dental caries.

- **Natural, Organic, or Synthetic Vitamins** - Beginning in the 1900's, vitamin and mineral supplements have exploded in the marketplace. Health claims have attempted to influence consumers to purchase "natural" or "organic" vitamins due to their supposed increased absorption and health benefits. These products compete with synthetic forms of vitamins by making false claims and are usually more expensive. In fact, there is no scientific evidence showing that the body uses natural or organic vitamins and minerals better than synthetic forms. The body does not recognize a natural or organic vitamin or mineral supplement any different than it would a synthetic form.

- **Time-Released Supplements** - Slowing vitamin-mineral supplement absorption was originally designed to allow their availability in the body for longer periods of time. Unfortunately, it turns out that the nutrients in time-released supplements are often more poorly absorbed. Some nutrients have also been found to be more toxic to certain body organs when in time-released forms than in similar doses of regular vitamin-mineral supplements. Therefore, the use of time-released supplements should be monitored or avoided if possible.

Answers to Vitamin and Mineral Questions

1. True. Taking a daily supplement will ensure adequate nutrient intake.

2. True. A variety of foods should encompass all necessary vitamins and minerals; however, a daily vitamin would never hurt if not exceeding the RDA.

3. False. A vitamin supplement may be taken in addition to a healthy diet. No vitamin supplement can replace the nutrients and fiber in healthy foods.

4. True. In cases of stress, increased energy needs, or lack of consumption of all food groups, a vitamin supplement is important to avoid deficiencies.

5. False. As long as you meet the RDA for vitamins and minerals, there is no need to double your daily intake.

6. False. Neither form is better than the other; however, if you are deficient in a specific nutrient, a single supplement may be more beneficial. On the other hand, if you want to ensure adequate vitamin and mineral intake throughout the day, a multivitamin would be more beneficial to you.

7. False. There is no evidence supporting this claim. All vitamins are recognized the same in the body no matter the source.

The chart below shows the USDA daily amounts. The vitamins and minerals with ** can be dangerous in excess amounts.

Nutrient	RDA males (31-50)	RDA females (31-50)
Fat Soluble Vitamins		
Vitamin A**	900 mcg RAE	700 mcg RAE
Beta-carotene**	none	none
Vitamin D**	5 mcg	5 mcg
Vitamin E	15 mg α-TE	15 mg α-TE
Vitamin K	120 mcg	90 mcg
Water Soluble Vitamins		
Vitamin B1	1.2 mg	1.1 mg
Vitamin B2	1.3 mg	1.1 mg
Niacin	16 mg NE	14 mg NE
Vitamin B6	1.3 mg	1.3 mg
Vitamin B12	2.4 mcg	2.4 mcg
Folic Acid	400 mcg DFE	400 mcg DFE
Biotin	30 mcg	30 mcg
Pantothenic Acid	5 mg	5 mg
Vitamin C	90 mg	75 mg

Nutrient	RDA males (31-50)	RDA females (31-50)
Minerals		
Calcium**	1000 mg	1000 mg
Chromium	35 mcg	25 mcg
Copper**	900 mcg	900 mcg
Iron**	8 mg	18 mg
Magnesium	420 mg	320 mg
Manganese	2.3 mg	1.8 mg
Molybdenum	45 mcg	45 mcg
Selenium	55 mcg	55 mcg
Zinc**	11 mg	8 mg

Review the following chart to see where you can obtain vitamins from your food

Vitamin A	*Vitamin C*	*Vitamin E*	*Vitamin D*
Tomatoes	Oranges	Almonds	Herring
Carrots	Red and Green Peppers	Sunflower oil	Salmon
Sweet Potatoes	Brussel Sprouts	Asparagus	Fort. Milk
Pumpkin	Papaya	Peanuts	Sardines

Vitamin K	*Thiamine*	*Riboflavin*	*Vitamin B6*
Spinach	Fortified Cereal	Beef Liver	Potato
Iceberg Lettuce	Pork chop	Fortified Cereal	Banana
Broccoli	Ham	Milk	White rice
Cabbage	Sunflower seeds	Yogurt	Chicken

Folate	*Vitamin B12*
Fortified dry cereal	Beef liver
Black-eyed peas	Clams
Lentils	Oysters
Spinach	Crab

SECTION 2

LOSING & MAINTAINING WEIGHT

WEIGHING YOUR BEST

"TO EAT IS A NECESSITY, BUT TO EAT INTELLIGENTLY IS AN ART."
- LA ROUCHEFOUCAULD

Forget about those commercials promising fast and easy weight loss. Losing weight is a process that takes time. And successful weight loss is not measured by how much you lose, but rather by how much you keep off and for how long. We feel there are three ingredients to success: motivation, commitment, and consistency. Not only must you really want to permanently lose weight, but you must commit to long term behavior changes and stick with them.

Spend some time before you begin a weight loss program and ask yourself why you have decided to lose weight. Identify at least three reasons and write them on an index card, notebook, or computer and reference them daily. You'll reinforce your decision to make permanent lifestyle changes. Learning new eating habits that are independent of others will make it easier for you to reach and maintain your goals.

As many of us know, weight gain comes easy. Since more than two-thirds of adults and more than one-third of children are overweight or obese, the 2010 Dietary Guidelines strongly urge Americans to eat less and get more active. A 2010 study in the Journal of the American Medical Association states that most Americans gain about 1.5 pounds a year from age 25 to 55. For many, the gradual weight gain with age is due to metabolism, genetics, hormones, less activity, less exercise, and an increase in calories. Even sleep habits play a role in what one weighs. The Sleep Medicine Program at the New York University School of Medicine suggests that the hormones leptin and ghrelin (affected by lack of sleep) may affect our drive to eat. Lower levels of leptin mean we don't feel satisfied after eating and higher levels of ghrelin increases appetite.

Dr. Kevin Hall at the National Institute of Diabetes and Digestive and Kidney Diseases reports that by just adding 10 calories daily over thirty years you can gain as much as 20 pounds. Ten calories is the equivalent to a stick a gum. In 2006, over 70% of Americans dieted. Yet studies have shown that most people do not maintain a weight loss. While diets usually dictate what to eat, they don't take into account food preferences, cultural habits, schedule, or lifestyle. Most dieters eventually get frustrated with all the restrictions that many commercial diets provide. They miss certain foods and find the restrictions impossible to maintain. They wind up "giving up" and returning to the original eating style - the one that contributed to weight gain in the first place! Our rule of thumb when choosing a diet plan is "Don't do anything while dieting that you can't do the rest of your life."

One of the best studies to date is from the National Weight Control Registry, co-founded in 1994 by Rena Wing, Professor of Psychiatry and Human Behavior at Brown University. It is the largest ongoing study of people that have not only lost weight, but more importantly, have kept it off. The study follows about 6,000 individuals who had lost at least 30 pounds and maintained the weight loss for at least 1 year. On average, participants kept it off for 6 years. As challenging as losing and maintaining weight loss can be, these individuals took a simple and practical approach by choosing behavior changes they could live with.

Common characteristics of "weight losers"

- Most had dieted before but were unable to keep the weight off.

- They used a combination of diet and exercise.

- About half got help by using a dietitian or joining Weight Watchers. Women liked having help, while men tended to go at it alone.

- Some counted calories; others counted fat grams.

- Many restricted high calorie foods like desserts or at least reduced the amounts they ate.

- Only a few used drastic measures such as liquid diets.

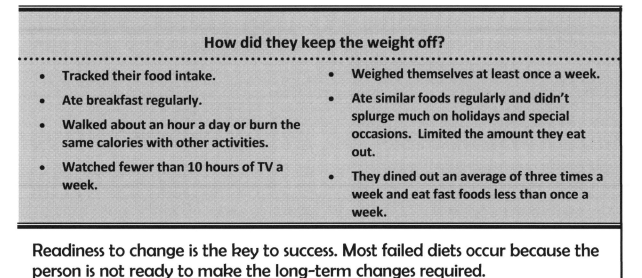

How did they keep the weight off?

- Tracked their food intake.
- Ate breakfast regularly.
- Walked about an hour a day or burn the same calories with other activities.
- Watched fewer than 10 hours of TV a week.

- Weighed themselves at least once a week.
- Ate similar foods regularly and didn't splurge much on holidays and special occasions. Limited the amount they eat out.
- They dined out an average of three times a week and eat fast foods less than once a week.

Readiness to change is the key to success. Most failed diets occur because the person is not ready to make the long-term changes required.

DETERMINING YOUR WEIGHT

There are different ways to determine what you should weigh. Height and weight tables are commonly used, but remember they do not take into account age, muscle mass, weight history, or genetics.

Get out the measuring tape to determine your waist circumference. Men should be no larger than 40 inches, and women 35 inches. An increase in 2 inches can raise the risk of metabolic syndrome by 17%. Visceral fat found deep inside the abdomen negatively impacts health. Most importantly, this fat is linked to insulin resistance, type 2 diabetes, hypertension, and heart disease. Weight loss can shrink the fat cells, allowing them to work correctly. Take a measurement at the smallest part of your waist and monitor this as you would your weight.

One of the most widely used methods by physicians and researchers is the Body Mass Index (BMI). BMI uses a formula that takes your height and weight into account. BMI is calculated by dividing a person's weight in kilograms by their height in meters squared. ($BMI=kg/m^2$). Don't worry about calculating it the table available has already done the math. To use the table, find your height in inches in the left-hand column. Move across the row to your weight. The number at the top of the column is your BMI.

The BMI is an indicator of body fat, which is closely related to risk of disease. Risk of disease is a phrase used to assess the possible future health consequences of an individual due to their current health status. A high disease risk is most often seen in overweight or obese individuals due to the fact that these individuals classically have the most health problems. Heart disease, stroke, cardiac arrhythmias, diabetes, hypertension, high cholesterol, and high triglycerides are a few examples of the unwanted health consequences associated with increased BMI and waist circumference. Therefore, it is important to maintain a normal BMI in order to lower your risk of disease and maintain optimal health.

An ideal BMI is between 18.5 and 24.9. As you can see in the following table, the weight category in this range is classified as normal, and the risk of disease is low. When the BMI climbs past the normal range and into the overweight and obese categories, the risk of disease greatly increases. On the other hand, when your BMI is below 18.5, you are considered underweight and although the risk of disease is low, other health consequences could result.

There are some limitations to the BMI calculation for certain individuals. For those who are athletes or have a large muscular build or frame, the BMI may overestimate the total body fat since it uses weight. Also, for the elderly or others who have depleted muscle mass, the BMI may underestimate the total body fat. Since everyone is built differently, BMI may not always be the best indicator of body fat. Waist circumference may be helpful. Remember, the risk of heart disease and other health problems increases with a waist circumference of over 40 inches in men and over 35 inches in women.

Determining Your Body Mass Index (BMI)

BMI (kg/m^2)	19	20	21	22	23	24	25	26	27	28	29	30	35	40
Height (in.)	Weight (lb.)													
58	91	96	100	105	110	115	119	124	129	134	138	143	167	191
59	94	99	104	109	114	119	124	128	133	138	143	148	173	198
60	97	102	107	112	118	123	128	133	138	143	148	153	179	204
61	100	106	111	116	122	127	132	137	143	148	153	158	185	211
62	104	109	115	120	126	131	136	142	147	153	158	164	191	218
63	107	113	118	124	130	135	141	146	152	158	163	169	197	225
64	110	116	122	128	134	140	145	151	157	163	169	174	204	232
65	114	120	126	132	138	144	150	156	162	168	174	180	210	240
66	118	124	130	136	142	148	155	161	167	173	179	186	216	247
67	121	127	134	140	146	153	159	166	172	178	185	191	223	255
68	125	131	138	144	151	158	164	171	177	184	190	197	230	262
69	128	135	142	149	155	162	169	176	182	189	196	203	236	270
70	132	139	146	153	160	167	174	181	188	195	202	207	243	278
71	136	143	150	157	165	172	179	186	193	200	208	215	250	286
72	140	147	154	162	169	177	184	191	199	206	213	221	258	294
73	144	151	159	166	174	182	189	197	204	212	219	227	265	302
74	148	155	163	171	179	186	194	202	210	218	225	233	272	311
75	152	160	168	176	184	192	200	208	216	224	232	240	279	319
76	156	164	172	180	189	197	205	213	221	230	238	246	287	328

Source: National Heart Lung & Blood Institute

Risk of Associated Disease According to BMI and Waist Size

BMI	Weight Category	Risk of Disease
18.5 or less	Underweight	Low
18.5 - 24.9	Normal	Low
25.0 - 29.9	Overweight	High
30.0 - 34.9	Obese	Very High
35.0 - 39.9	Obese	Very High
40 or greater	Morbid Obese	Extremely High

WHAT IF I AM AT HIGH RISK FOR DISEASE?

Perform the waist circumference assessment to determine if you are over the recommended measurement. Once BMI and waist circumference have been evaluated, consider your other risk factors.

If you have any of these risk factors, in addition to a high BMI and/or waist circumference, become proactive in improving your health. Generally, losing weight is the first step to lowering your BMI, waist circumference, and risk of disease. Studies show that even a 10% weight loss will reduce your risk of disease significantly.

Risk factors include the following:

- High blood pressure
- High LDL-cholesterol level
- Low HDL-cholesterol level
- High triglycerides level
- Diabetes
- Family history of heart disease
- Physical inactivity
- Cigarette smoking
- Excess alcohol consumption

HOW MUCH TO EAT?

We are all different when it comes to the number of calories needed throughout the day. Age, gender, physical activity, and metabolism all play a role. As a general rule, men need more calories than women due to larger size and muscle mass. Also, as we age, our calorie needs decrease significantly due to a slower metabolism. It's important to match your energy intake (calories) with energy expenditure (physical activity) to avoid gaining weight.

We think knowing your daily calorie needs is one of the most important pieces of information when trying to lose or maintain weight. Yet, according to a survey by the International Food Information Council a mere 12 percent of Americans know how many calories they need in a day. Studies have shown that most people underestimate their calorie intake by as much as 25 percent.

Here's a simple formula to help you estimate your caloric requirement: take your current weight (in pounds) and multiply it by 12 and you'll have an estimate of about how many calories you need to maintain your current weight. Dr. Kevin Hall and his researchers discovered that a 250 calories a day reduction in calories leads to weight loss of about 25 pounds over three years. About half of that loss happens in the first year. Remember, when you've reached your weight goal your calorie needs may not be much more than what you were using to lose weight.

Regardless of age or gender, if you are a very active individual, your calorie needs will be higher to maintain weight than those who are not active. Most moderately active women will lose weight consuming about 1500 calories, men about 2,000 calories. Try to trim 250 to 500 calories off your day. Spend thirty minutes exercising and you'll burn about 200 calories. Choosemyplate.gov provides a calorie calculator based upon your age, weight, and activity level.

THE SCALE: FRIEND OR FOE

Weighing regularly can actually enhance your weight loss efforts. The scale provides immediate feedback. You'll see changes in your weight from overeating and be able to adjust your calories immediately. You'll also identify pounds that come and go possibly due to fluid shifts, exercise, sodium intake, or hormonal changes. By checking your weight regularly (at least once or twice a week) you can determine if the calorie level you've selected is providing a consistent weight loss of anywhere from three to eight pounds per month. Also, if you are always hungry and find yourself obsessing about food, you've probably reduced your calories too much. A steady slow weight loss of 3 to 6 lbs per month provides the opportunity to make permanent behavior changes. Once you reach your weight goal. the scale can keep you on track and eliminate any surprise weight gain. If you find yourself up a few pounds you can quickly assess your eating and exercise and adjust if necessary. Consult a registered dietitian in your area for a complete and accurate breakdown of your calorie needs. Check www.eatright.org for the name of a local registered dietitian or ask your physician for the name of someone he refers to.

BE HONEST, KEEP A FOOD LOG

We can't emphasize enough the importance of keeping a log or food diary. A food log helps keep you honest. Recent studies show that the best predictor of weight loss is logging what you eat. In fact, people who track their calories lose twice as much weight as those who don't.

Food logs should include: food, portions, calories, time, place, activity, and feelings. Tedious as it may seem, it's worth the effort to keep a log when you are trying to lose weight. You'll identify the 'why's and "what's" of your eating. You'll also discover if your life is booby trapped with opportunities to overeat. Remember visual/external cues are the strongest cues to eat. By logging, you can create an eating environment that makes it easier to be successful in a busy world. Here are tips we use:

1. Don't purchase high calorie foods that are tempting to eat.

2. Do purchase low calorie snacks you enjoy.

3. Store tempting foods so they are not visible; out of sight, out of mind.

4. Don't serve meals family style; you'll avoid seconds.

5. Put fresh fruit on the counter or table rather than the refrigerator.

6. Portion snacks ahead of time according to your calorie budget.

7. Use smaller plates, bowls, and glasses.

8. Read labels for calorie information.

9. Dejunk your cabinets and drawers.

10. Include your favorite foods; it is the frequency and quantity that counts.

Make sure your food log is portable and keep it within reach at all times. Any notebook will do, or pick up a food diary from your local bookstore. Subtotal after meals and snacks so you know how many calories you've spent and what you have left. With today's technology, some individuals keep their calories logged on blackberries, iPhones, or laptop computers. The free *Lose It* application and *My Fitness Plan* can be downloaded to an iPhone, making calorie counting easy. The book Calorie King can be used or the website : www.calorieking.com. The book *Bite It & Write It: A Guide to Keeping Track of What You Eat & Drink* is another food journal available. An example of a food log can be found in appendix A.

BALANCE YOUR BUDGET

Your calorie quota can be thought of as a budget of calories, similar to a checking account. You have a certain amount to "spend" each day, and like any budget, you must adjust your expenditures to stay within the limit. Favorite foods that might be high in calories are often perceived as "not allowed". By counting calories no foods are forbidden and dieters can adjust calories to include foods and beverages they might otherwise avoid. You'll eliminate the guilt that accompanies eating high calorie items and improve your relationship with food.

Subtotal calories after meals and snacks so you have a running account of how many calories you've spent and what you have left. If you find yourself eating more at lunch than you had originally planned, you can balance your calorie budget by eating less at dinner. Avoid the mindset that if a food is "good for you" it doesn't count. All foods have calories, so they all matter. Even excessive amounts of fruits or beverages can interfere with losing weight. A Café Mocha from Starbucks will cost you 400 calories; a Caffe Americano, only 15. You may have to spend close to an hour exercising to work off this high calorie beverage.

Recording what you eat helps identify eating patterns. Avoid grazing. Most grazers never feel hungry and lose track of how much they've eaten. Meal skippers shift most of their calories to the evening. The end result: Not much time left to burn off those calories!

Common characteristics of chronically overweight individuals
• They eat the majority of their calories in the evening • They skip breakfast and sometimes lunch • They snack after dinner

Americans are notorious for eating the majority of their calories at dinner. Work days and commutes have gotten longer and so dinner is often later. Think calories in vs. calories out. If you're active you should eat. As your day winds down it makes sense that you require less calories. This simple change can make a big difference in what you weigh. You wouldn't run your car on empty all day, and then fill it up at night only to park it.

Look at your meals and remember this adage
Eat breakfast like a king Lunch like a prince and Dinner like a pauper

IT'S MORE THAN WHAT YOU EAT

By writing how you feel when you eat (happy, stressed, tired) you will also identify the connection between your mood and what, when, why, and how much you eat. This link will allow you to work out behaviors that cause you to eat the wrong foods, the wrong amounts, and at the wrong times. By identifying foods you eat when you feel a certain way you can substitute lower calorie food. The temporary "feel good" that comes with high calorie foods is no more than a quick fix. You can short circuit an impulse to eat by identifying feelings or activities that led to the over eating. You can then substitute a different activity. Use an activity that's suitable for that "feeling/mood". If you're tired, take a short nap, or distract yourself by doing yoga or taking a walk.

Discover if your home or work place is "booby trapped" with tempting foods. You may need to do some spring cleaning in your cabinets and drawers and fill the candy jar with low calorie, tasty snacks.

Food logs identify "unnecessary eating" allowing you to reconsider whether you want to spend your calories on a particular food.

Food Log Tips

1. Carry your food log with you at all times.

2. Record everything you eat and drink.

3. Record the amounts you eat and the calories provided.

4. Record as soon after eating as you can.

5. Record the time of day or night you eat.

6. Record how you feel when you eat.

7. Record your daily physical activity.

8. Keep a running count of your calories by subtotaling the calories after each meal so you know what's left in your budget.

9. Record your weight as often as you need, e.g. daily, weekly, to see the relationship between your calorie intake and your weight.

As an example, see the food diary at the end of this section. This can be copied several times or loaded onto a computer to track.

THE FULLNESS FACTOR

Individual foods have what we refer to as a satiety index, or "fullness factor." The satiety index of a food refers to the level of fullness and how long that feeling stays with you after eating. The three major nutrients that make up food (carbohydrate, protein, and fat) affect how long you remain satisfied (or satiated) after eating. Foods with protein, fiber, and water keep you feeling full longer. Dr. Susanne Holt, Australian researcher at the University of Sydney, compared a variety of foods to determine their satiety index. Her research reported in 1995 had a few surprises. Apples, oranges, all bran, porridge, potatoes, popcorn, and white fish were rated the highest for satiety. Cookies, cakes, croissants, and peanuts rated a lower score for fullness. So, if you find yourself hungry in the middle of the afternoon, choose a snack that will prevent you from being ravenous by dinnertime .

Discover your snack satiety index. First, determine the amount of calories you can spend on a snack. Most women should keep snacks around 100 to 150 calories, men 150 to 200 calories. Choose snacks that you enjoy within that calorie level. Determine your satiety index by tracking when you get hungry after eating those snacks.

High Satiety Snacks

- 1 slice of cheese
- 15 almonds
- large apple
- ½ cup of cottage cheese

- no-fat yogurt
- 1 ounce of chocolate
- 3 cups of popcorn
- 1 cup vegetable soup

Avoid meal-skipping patterns!

- **Grab breakfast.** Make breakfast a priority. Whether running to make an early appointment, dropping kids off at school, or catching a plane, take time to eat or drink something nutritious. Make sure to include at least 7 grams of protein. Though the morning is usually a rush, there are plenty of breakfast foods that are quick, easy to prepare, or even portable. Planning is the key.

- **Break for lunch.** Eat a lunch with at least 300 calories. Pack a lunch when possible if you're on the run. It takes only a few extra minutes in the morning, or the night before, to pull together a nutritious meal. If you spend a lot of time in the car, keep a cooler packed with water, fruit, cheese, and other portable foods. Reference the calorie information at fast food restaurants if necessary. If you eat lunch out, try to eat dinner at home. Or, if your schedule includes dinner out, try to pack a lunch.

- **Plan for dinner.** Think ahead to dinner and plan for the right expenditure of calories. Have foods available that can be quickly prepared. There are many cookbooks with 30 minutes or less recipes. Watch your portions.

If eating later in the evening, try appetizers or splitting a meal rather than a large meal late at night. Shift more of your calories earlier in the day to avoid being hungry.

A good rule is: *The later the dinner, the lesser the calories.* Plan and you can keep your calorie budget balanced!

WEIGHT GAIN AND MENOPAUSE

The weight gain that accompanies menopause can be frustrating and seems to sneak up on most women. During this time women can gain as much as 15 pounds, and most weight settles in the middle leaving most women wondering what happened to their waist.   Without a doubt, body shape is changing and fat distribution shifts from arms, legs, and hips to the abdomen. Visceral fat also increases during menopause. We know that excess fat, particularly in the middle, can increase the risk for stroke, cardiovascular disease, diabetes, and metabolic syndrome. Hormones are in a state of flux—estrogen declining and testosterone increasing—influencing the distribution of fat.

Be proactive. Metabolism also decreases during this time, so women need to be prepared to review and adjust their calorie intake if gaining weight. You may need to decrease your daily calories by 200 to 300 calories. Weighing regularly (at least weekly) can prevent weight from sneaking up on you. Many adults decrease their protein intake as they age. But researchers are finding that more protein may be necessary for the older adult, especially protein foods that contain the amino acid leucine. According to researcher Christos Katsanos at Arizona State University, more amino acids are needed to stimulate protein synthesis (building new muscle). Animal proteins (meat, poultry, dairy, fish, and eggs) are the best sources. Whey also contains leucine. He suggests aiming for at least 20 grams of protein at each meal. Spread the protein over the course of the day and eat a source of protein after a workout. The U.S. dietary guidelines recommend 0.8 grams of protein (or more) for every 2.2 pounds of body weight. For example, a person who weighs 150 pounds should take in about 56 grams of protein a day. A 4 ounce chicken breast has about 28 grams, a glass of milk 8 grams and a Greek yogurt about 13 grams.

Stay active. Increasing activity is just as important as reducing calories to avoid weight gain. We begin losing about a quarter pound of muscle each year beginning in our late 30's or early 40's. More muscle means burning more calories. In fact, we have found that women who have a regular exercise program (at least 30 minutes daily) gain the least amount of weight. The Journal of the American Medical Association reports that women need 60 minutes of moderate-intensity exercise daily to avoid weight gain as they move from their twenties and thirties into middle age. Researchers from the University of Pittsburg also found that individuals avoided weight gain by following a diet of 1300 calories and by doing exercise that burns 1000 to 1500 calories per day. Weight strengthening exercises builds new muscle, slows muscle loss, and increases bone density. This is especially important for the menopausal woman whose body is undergoing so many changes. A combination of aerobic and weight strengthening is best. This might be a good time to visit with a registered dietitian and a personal trainer to develop a program that's just right for you.

Tips and Tricks of the Trade that we use to avoid weight gain

1. Know the calories you require to lose or maintain weight.

2. Eat a consistent diet most days.

3. Don't skip meals.

4. Stay active. Exercise at least 30 minutes a day.

5. Weigh yourself regularly.

6. Avoid allowing a small weight gain to turn into more.

No matter what your age, losing, and maintaining weight is a complicated process and requires vigilance. A recent study published in American Journal of Clinical Nutrition found that among a group of women, (average age 58) who had lost 25 pounds, in many of those who regained weight, the pounds returned as fat mass rather than muscle mass. Keep in mind these women were sedentary.

We find many chronic dieters have lost confidence in their ability to sustain a weight loss. Some perceive food as the enemy; others use it as comfort when under stress, bored, feeling anxious, or sad. Develop a good relationship with food and exercise. Never take the "all or nothing" approach. Small changes in calories and activity can result in weight loss that is permanent. Remember too, that a good weight loss program is comprehensive and is provided by experts. If you need help tackling a weight problem contact a registered dietitian in your area.

The items below are reviews from Sarah Krieger, MPH, RD, LDN, of the top-rated free iPhone apps for weigh management from the Academy of Nutrition and Dietetics website.

- <u>Calorie Counter:</u> Tracks food, exercise, weight and all the nutrients listed on a Nutrition Label. Includes daily inspirational articles, healthy recipes, and an easy-to-understand help section. Rating: 4 stars
- <u>Calorie Counter & Diet Tracker by MyFitness Pal:</u> Tracks a combination of fitness goals and nutrition analysis features to help you lose weight. Rating: 4.5 stars
- <u>Calorie Counter: Diets & Activities:</u> Features a classic food diary that tracks calories, water, fitness and the time each food item is consumed and an option to create your own diet and physical activity plan and an integrated body tracker. Rating: 4 stars
- <u>Calorie Tracker by Livestrong.com:</u> Food and fitness diary designed to help you achieve your diet and nutrition goals, whether you want to lose, maintain or gain weight. Rating: 4 stars
- <u>Lose it!:</u> Keeps track of foods you eat with this detailed food database: primarily for people wanting to lose weight. Rating: 3 stars
- <u>Sparkpeople Food and Fitness Tracker:</u> Fitness and food tracker for people looking to lose a half-pound to 2 pound per week or to maintain weight. Rating: 4 stars

FAD DIETS

Fad Diet Questions: Test your knowledge of the most recent "fad" diets by answering <u>True</u> or <u>False</u> to the questions below.

1. Most fad diets are the same by reducing caloric intake as part of the diet.
2. I can choose any fad diet to help me lose weight, and I will see weight loss that will stay off for a very long time.
3. All fad diets are safe to try, and there are no consequences except for weight loss.
4. Incorporating exercise is an indicator of the safety of a fad diet.
5. A diet that incorporates more than 300 mg cholesterol daily will allow me to lose weight faster.
6. Low carbohydrate and more protein intake will give me the energy to exercise.

Promises, promises, weight loss claims that seem too good to be true. That's one thing that fad diets have in common. Fad diets have been around for decades. The seventies gave us the Atkins diet, high in protein and fat. We used liquid protein diets, where daily calorie intake was as low as 400 calories. Very overweight individuals enrolled in these liquid fast programs, often losing as much as 100 pounds. Most regained the weight.

Fad diets come and go. Atkins has resurged in interest over the past few years, but like our patients in the seventies and eighties, most individuals stick with the diet for a few months and then return to their old eating style. We find that when fad diets deprive dieters of a certain nutrient (carbohydrate in this case) or a certain food group, the desire for these foods increase.

We can't talk about fad diets without first discussing why fad diets are such an obsession in the United States.   Obesity has become a major health threat in America with two out of every three U.S. adults either overweight or obese. With obesity comes great health risks. One of the greatest risks of obesity is diabetes, accounting for one out of every ten health care dollars spent in the United States.   Some companies are working to reduce this risk by encouraging their employees to lose weight and maintain a healthy lifestyle. These attempts are leading to reduced health risks and reduced health insurance premiums.

If you have attempted a fad diet, you are not alone.   Every year millions of people attempt to lose weight with diet programs, or fad diets, encouraged by popular culture.   Most are as silly as their name.   Take for instance the Cabbage Soup diet. It promises weight loss stating that vegetables and fruits can burn fat.   Another new trend is a gluten-free diet. This diet is designed for those with celiac disease, wheat allergy, or wheat insensitivity. Celiac disease is a serious autoimmune disease that causes the flattening of the finger -like villi of the small intestine. A gluten-free diet can reverse the gastrointestinal symptoms including diarrhea, bloating, abdominal pain, and gas.

A gluten-free diet is not harmful for individuals who do not need it, but it is difficult to follow, costly, and can lead to vitamin, iron, and fiber deficiencies if you are not working with a registered dietitian who will help you design a healthy eating plan.

Many gluten-free products can also be higher in carbohydrate, sugar, fat, and calories than their normal counterparts. This can make weight reduction more difficult. If individuals lose weight on a gluten-free diet, returning to a diet with gluten can cause initial gastrointestinal symptoms that will eventually go away.

We wish dieting was easy! Unfortunately, these trendy diets are not supported by the medical community and can actually increase the public's risk of developing health problems. Although most fad diets work initially, over time you most likely see the weight creep back. Explanations include lifestyle, food behaviors, and food preferences. When the weight is off, life is good and the former eating patterns return, which caused the weight gain in the first place.

How many times have you and your significant other tried a diet together, and the other person lost more weight? Researchers have found a genetic reason for this frustrating point. Interleukin Genetics has identified three genes that can predict weight loss: genes ABP2, ADRB2, and PPAR-gamma. Studies of 133 women have shown that when certain diets were paired with certain genotypes, the appropriately paired women lost 3% more weight than those who weren't appropriately paired. Researchers conceded that obesity had more to do with environment than genotype, though they agreed genotype determined whether a person responded more favorably to a low fat or low carbohydrate diet.

If the fad diets you've tried don't include your favorite foods or match your eating style, weight loss will be difficult to maintain. The National Weight Control Registry is a database comprised of nearly 3,000 successful dieters. It gives us wonderful insight about what works when trying to lose weight. This registry was maintained from 1993-1997. Its participants lost an average of 66 pounds, and then maintained a 30-pound weight loss for over 5.5 years.

> Lifestyle changes, not short-term dietary changes, make the difference.

What did the experts find from this information? They identified key behavioral changes that enabled participants to successfully maintain weight loss including:

- Reduced calorie intake
- Reduced fat intake
- Increased physical activity

Other weight maintenance programs have also shown that individuals who aren't deprived of favorite high-calorie foods, but instead watch portion sizes, have a better success rate. These participants successfully maintained their weight loss because they did not view their dietary changes as temporary. These individuals were not waiting for the diet to end so they could return to overindulgence. Lifestyle changes, not short-term dietary changes, made the difference.

Fad diets can be risky for individuals with certain health conditions. Fad diets have also been found to place individuals at risk of coronary disease, cancer, gout, kidney stones, osteoporosis, keto-breath, fainting, dizziness, and high blood pressure. As registered dietitians with combined clinical experience of over 60 years, we have seen all of these medical problems resulting from inappropriate dieting methods.

When starting a diet plan, consider the following

1. Diets that promise a quick fix or make claims that are too good to be true should be questioned. Losing weight is not an easy process. If the plan promises quick results, it probably will not work in the long run.
2. Diets should not exclude food groups or tout particular foods as being "wonder" foods and others as being harmful.
3. For many years, the United States Department of Agriculture has stressed the importance of eating a variety of foods from each of the main food groups. By doing this, you increase your chances of obtaining the nutrients that your body needs. A helpful way to measure the safety of a new fad diet is to see what reputable health organizations say about it. These groups include the Academy of Nutrition and Dietetics, American Medical Association, American Heart Association, and the American Cancer Society.

Insure the diet plan being considered is nutritionally adequate, by using the following checklist

- Does the diet supply at least 25 grams of fiber each day?
- Does the diet contain at least five servings of fruit and vegetables daily?
- Does the diet provide less than 300 mg of cholesterol each day?
- Does the diet supply less than 10% of calories from saturated fat daily?

- Does the diet stress exercise as a component?
- Does the diet contain adequate carbohydrates to allow an individual to exercise safely?
- Does the diet specify the carbohydrate, protein, fat, types of fat, mineral, and vitamin contents to ensure that it meets the Recommended Dietary Allowance?

Lose weight and keep it off with these healthy behaviors

1. Increase the amounts of fruits, vegetables, non-fat dairy products, grains, and legumes you eat daily. These nutrient dense foods pack a lot of nutrition without the calories!
2. Reduce calorie-dense foods high in fat and refined carbohydrates such as: cookies, desserts, bagels, crackers, chips, fries, pizza, and candy.
3. Incorporate exercise as a component of your weight loss attempts.
4. Avoid eating your biggest meal late in the evening. Have a cut off time, limit or avoid eating after a certain hour, e.g., 8 p.m.

Type of Diet	Total Calories	Fat grams (% calories)	Carb grams (% calories)	Protein grams (% calories)	Nutrition Adequacy
Typical American Diet	2200	85 (35%)	275 (50%)	82.5 (15%)	
High Fat Low-Carbohydrate Diet · Dr. Atkins Diet · Zone Diet · Sugar Busters · Protein Power	1414	96 (60%) Fat Level Range: 35-65%	35 (10%)	105 (30%)	Low in several nutrients: Vitamins A, B6, D, E, thiamin, folate, calcium, magnesium, iron, zinc, potassium and dietary fiber. This type of diet also contains excess amounts of total fat, saturated fat, and dietary cholesterol. Nutritional supplementation is highly recommended.
Moderate Fat Diet · USDA Food Guide Pyramid · DASH Diet · American Diabetic Association · Weight Watchers · Jenny Craig	1450	40 (25%) Fat Level Range: 21-34%	218 (60%)	54 (15%)	Usually a nutritionally balanced eating plan assuming the dieter eats a variety of foods from all food categories. However, limiting certain food categories can lead to deficiencies in certain nutrients especially calcium, iron and zinc.
Low- and Very Low-Fat Diet · Volumetrics · Dean Ornish's Eat More, Weigh Less · New Pritikin Program	1450	20 (13%) Fat Level varies: 10-20%	235-271 (70%)	54-72 (17%)	Deficient in zinc and vitamin B12 due to infrequent meat consumption. Additionally, this type of diet can be inadequate in vitamin E, a nutrient found in oils, nuts, and other foods rich in fat.

*Source: Reprinted with permission from, Freedman, M., King, J. and Kennedy, E. Popular Diets: A Scientific Review. J of Obesity Research. 2001: Supplement 1.

Answers to Fad Diet Questions

1. True
2. False. You will lose weight with most fad diets, but you probably won't maintain the weight loss.
3. False. Fad diets have been found to place some individuals at risk of coronary disease, cancer, gout, kidney stones, osteoporosis, keto-breath, fainting, dizziness, and high blood pressure.
4. True
5. False. Carbohydrate converts to glucose in the body, which is the main source of energy for the body, especially the brain.   Low carbohydrate intake does not allow you to obtain the necessary energy to allow for safe exercise.

DETOX DIETS

The first thing that comes to mind when you hear the word "Detox" might be a treatment for alcohol or drug dependence. It can also refer to drugs, herbs, and other methods of removing diet and environmental toxins from the body. A detox diet involves the consumption of foods that help to eliminate harmful dietary, environmental, and other poisons which can aid in the improved function of the liver, lymphatic system, and kidneys.

The detox diet has come back into vogue. Detox is short for "detoxification," which is typically the body's natural process of eliminating toxins from the body. Detox diets try to imitate what the body does naturally, but these diets are often not safe or effective.

Toxins are harmful products to body tissues and are changed to less harmful compounds and excreted through stool or urine through detoxification. Toxins are made by the body as a result of normal body functions. For example, normal protein breakdown produces ammonia which is then converted to urea and excreted in the urine. Other toxic materials include:

There are a number of detox diets being advocated, and their characteristics are

- Generally a short-term diet where weight loss is not the primary goal.

- Include plans that minimize the chemicals ingested by using only organic foods.

- Encourage foods that provide vitamins, nutrients, and antioxidants that are necessary to the body for detoxification.

- Include foods that are high in fiber and water that will eliminate toxins by increasing the frequency of bowel movements and urination.

cigarette smoke, pesticides, household cleaners, drugs, pollution, or food additives.

Many individuals are seeking out the use of detox diets because they believe that the chemicals we consume can be deposited in the fat cells in our bodies. They believe their diets are lacking in proper nutrients, impairing the body's natural ability to remove chemicals leading to a build-up of toxins in the body. This build-up is thought to lead to illness which has been linked to hormonal imbalance, impaired immune function, poor skin, muscle pain, or bad breath. They fail to explain how a diet rich in fruits, vegetables, and unprocessed foods will allow the body to naturally detoxify these chemicals.

Detox risks include

- Nutritional deficiency
- Headache
- Diarrhea leading to dehydration and electrolyte loss
- Constipation if not drinking enough water with increased fiber

- Fatigue
- Weight loss
- Irritability
- Acne
- Hunger leading to overeating when a regular diet is resumed

Proponents may even offer labs where they can assess urine, stool, blood, and liver function. Many physicians and dietitians do not recognize these labs, do not endorse them, and question the validity of the results.

Remember that individuals prescribing these diets should be doing so only with the advice of a physician. Individuals should be visiting their physician for signs of fatigue, indigestion, cough, etc. that could be sign of serious illness.

Individuals who should not attempt a detox diet include

- Pregnant or nursing women
- Children
- Eating disordered individuals

- Those with chronic disease such as diabetes, thyroid disease, kidney disease
- Those with cancer
- Those with terminal illness

GLYCEMIC INDEX DIET FOR WEIGHT LOSS

Though the Glycemic Index (GI) is a new nutrition buzzword, it has been around for decades. In 1981, Dr. David Jenkins from the University of Toronto discovered that even though foods may have identical carbohydrate content, their effect on blood sugar may be quite different. This discovery is known as the GI of foods, and it is a useful tool for people with diabetes to help control their blood sugars. The number associated with GI represents the rate at which carbohydrate in a food raises blood sugar after eating.

There are many factors involved in the rise of blood sugar after eating, such as cooking time, processing of foods, ripeness, fiber, protein, and fat content. Even activity level can affect the rate at which a high carbohydrate food may affect the rise in blood sugar. For most individuals without diabetes, the GI of foods is not a concern. In fact, according to the American Diabetes Association, portion sizes will affect a rise in glucose level and the amount of weight gain.

There is a list of foods available, based on research, which rank foods measured by a rise in blood sugar. The index compares foods to glucose, which has a 100% numerical value. What's important to know is that some low calorie, healthy foods may have a high glycemic index, e.g., boiled potato (78). Some low glycemic index foods may include foods that provide little nutrition and lots of calories, e.g., chocolate (40). Ice cream has a lower glycemic index (51) than brown rice (68) and rice crackers (87). We know if ice cream is eaten with each meal, it will most likely result in a weight increase. Therefore, it's still important to look at the nutrient level and portion size of the food when you are dieting.

The American Diabetes Association provides the following GI ranking of foods based on how quickly they raise blood glucose levels. The reference foods, white bread or glucose, have a GI of 100

Low GI Foods (55 or less)

- 100% stone-ground whole wheat or pumpernickel bread
- Oatmeal (rolled or steel-cut), oat bran, muesli
- Pasta, converted rice, barley, bulgur
- Sweet potato, corn, yam, lima/butter beans, peas, legumes and lentils
- Most fruits, non-starchy vegetables and carrots

Medium GI (56-69)

- Whole wheat, rye and pita bread
- Quick oats
- Brown, wild or basmati rice, couscous

High GI (70 or more)

- White bread or bagel
- Corn flakes, puffed rice, bran flakes, instant oatmeal
- Short grain white rice, rice pasta, macaroni and cheese from mix
- Russet potato, pumpkin
- Pretzels, rice cakes, popcorn, saltine crackers
- Melons and pineapple

More recently the GI has been recommended as a weight loss diet. Insulin is an anabolic (weight gain) hormone. Some individuals who have extra insulin being produced may store extra calories that can easily result in weight gain. Most of us eat a variety of foods that include high glycemic index foods, e.g., mashed potatoes, bread, corn flakes, etc. Weight loss from following a low glycemic diet usually results from eliminating a variety of foods and therefore reducing the overall calories. Most individuals who follow the low G.I. diet hoping to lose weight will wind up eliminating high calorie foods—e.g., desserts, breads, pastas—and lose weight.

As we've said before, weight loss occurs after reducing the daily calorie intake so there isn't anything magical about a low glycemic index diet when used for weight loss purposes. We stick by our motto "don't do anything while dieting that you can't do the rest of your life."

EXERCISE

Work out your Exercise knowledge by answering <u>True</u> or <u>False</u> to the following questions:

1. Schedule conflicts and time constraints are two major obstacles that keep you from participating in a regular exercise program.

2. To reduce the risk of chronic disease, Americans should aim for at least 30 minutes of physical activity 3-5 times per week.

3. Health clubs are a great place for everyone, especially busy people, to exercise.

4. If you schedule exercise into your work week, you are more likely to exercise.

5. Activity and exercise can have a significant impact on an individual's weight.

6. Wanting to lose weight and not being willing to exercise is okay.

7. Planning ways to incorporate exercise into the day shows a willingness to make change.

8. Working mothers have no time to exercise and cannot easily increase their activity level.

What's the latest on exercise? The Surgeon General has indicated even moderate amounts of activity can improve health. The 2010 Dietary Guidelines recommend at least 30 minutes of exercise daily. Exercise and our overall daily level of activity can play a big part in our health and what we weigh. Dr. Peter Katzmarzyk, epidemiologist at the Pennington Biomedical Research Center in Baton Rouge, Louisiana, found that people who spend most of their day sitting have a higher mortality rate than people who don't.

In fact, researchers at Mayo Clinic have given "fidgeters" a reprieve. They studied a small group of individuals who overate for two months. They tracked not only their fat storage but also the amount of calories burned during normal activity. The fidgeters (those that moved more) gained less fat then those that did not. So, fidgeting counts. Mayo Clinic has coined this activity as NEAT, nonexercise activity thermogenesis. NEAT is defined as the energy you burn doing activities that are not formal exercise. So forget sitting still and instead look for opportunities to move around during the day. Take phone calls standing up or pace as you talk. Stand, stretch, bend; anything is better than sitting still. Advanced technology, long days at work, and sitting at computers all day can affect our health and weight.

Is body image a concern? A recent study in the Journal of Health Psychology shows that those individuals that exercised, even without the usual benefits of weight loss and increased muscle mass, had improved their body image. Even memory and the ability to learn seem to be improved with exercise, say researchers at University of Illinois in a 2006 study.

For young adults, being physically active is an investment in the future. Let's face it, if you're reluctant to regularly exercise now, beginning a program later in life will not be any easier. Recent studies show that the fragility that comes with getting older can be reduced significantly through exercise. In fact, Dr. Cheryl Phillips, president of the American Geriatric Society states, "Physical activity is more powerful than any medication a senior can take." That should be enough to get you started!

What's the obstacle to consistently exercising? For most it is time constraints; for others the couch or computer fills our spare time. Usually the major challenge is fitting exercise into an already busy schedule. Here are 10 good reasons to inspire you to exercise.

Reasons to Exercise		
1. Helps you maintain weight	6.	Promotes healthy bones
2. Helps you lose weight	7.	Increases muscle mass
3. Improves blood circulation	8.	Reduces stress
4. Improves blood pressure	9.	Decreases your risk for diabetes
5. Improves mood	10.	May allow you to eat more

BEFORE STARTING EXERCISE

Depending on your age, health status, and level of fitness, you may want to obtain clearance from you doctor before starting an exercise program to ensure your safety and know your risks.

Check with your doctor before exercising if you have any of the following health issues

- cardiovascular disease
- musculoskeletal problems
- neurological abnormalities
- cardiac, pulmonary, or metabolic disease - you should begin your exercise in a medically supervised environment

SELECTING AN EXERCISE

Exercise, like a pair of shoes, has to be a good fit to work. Too many times individuals choose an exercise program that does not fit their lifestyle or can only be done certain times of the year. If you are just starting to exercise, you probably want to start with activities that are not too intense, such as walking or biking. Walking, running, or biking when the weather is warm is great, but when the temperature drops, so often does the exercise routine. If you decide on an outdoor activity, have a back-up plan for bad weather. Invest in indoor exercise equipment if possible, such as a treadmill or stationary bike. Treadmills allow you to walk and run and also give you the advantage of controlling the intensity of your workout with speed and incline. Spinning and dance classes are fun indoor activities.

If you can't afford equipment or don't have the room, take advantage of exercise programs on television, video, or DVD. If on the road or on vacation, pack some music and practice your new moves in a hotel room. If your trip includes hills or beaches, plan on hiking or walking. See the city you're visiting on foot or bike. An early morning run or walk means you beat the crowds. Take an after-dinner walk to burn off some of the evening calories.

Tips for Scheduling Exercise

- Measure your activity with a pedometer (a device you wear that counts your steps throughout the day and translates into miles or kilometers).
- Keep exercise clothes with you in the car so you can stop at the gym whenever you have time.
- Find opportunities to exercise if you find yourself waiting for an appointment or a child at an activity.
- When traveling, try to find hotels that have a fitness room or pool.
- Partner with a colleague or friend and exercise together.
- Bypass the elevator and use the stairs when possible.
- Avoid planning exercises that are too time-consuming for your schedule.

At the end of the chapter you can find a list of various activities to let you know how many calories you are burning. This can also assist you when trying to decide on a workout that will fit your lifestyle and fitness goals. You can also check how many calories you burn at http://www.clevelandclinic.orghealth/interactive/burned.asp, by using their easy to use calorie calculator.

Health Clubs—Pros and Cons

Pro's	Con's
Easy to find: Health clubs can be found in neighborhoods, in the building we live in, and sometimes even in the workplace.	*Price:* Membership can be expensive, so before you join make sure you will make use of it.
Variety of Equipment: Health clubs have a wide variety of both cardiovascular and strength-training equipment.	*Travel:* Sometimes the additional travel time to and from a health club may not be realistic for a really busy person.
Group exercise classes: Some clubs offer classes that can be more fun than exercising alone. Examples are yoga, kickboxing, spinning, and dance.	*Waiting:* During peak times, you may find yourself waiting for popular pieces of fitness equipment.
Personal trainers: Most clubs have trainers available to assist in individualizing a program that's right for you.	*Time:* Exercising before or during the work day requires extra time to shower and change.
Socializing: Health clubs are a great way to meet people and even find an exercise buddy.	
Locations: Some clubs allow you to work out at any of their facilities across the country, which can be convenient when traveling.	

PERSONAL TRAINERS

If you decide a personal trainer is right for you, make sure to find one that is certified and experienced, since there are no legal regulations for personal trainers. Certification should come from a well known organization such as the Cooper Institute, the National Academy of Sports Medicine, the American College of Sports Medicine, the American Council on Exercise, or the National Strength and Conditioning Association. You can also look for a certified trainer in the American College of Sports Medicine (ACSM) database. Check online at www.ideafit.com for a Personal Fitness Trainer (PFT) or on the ACSM website: www.acsm.org.   Before choosing a personal trainer, observe them working with other clients or ask friends for a referral. Some trainers may even give you a free session to see if you like it.

A trainer can help evaluate your body composition as well as put together a complete program that includes cardiovascular fitness, flexibility, and strength-training.   If you have a history of medical complications such as heart attacks, diabetes, or injuries, make sure to talk to your doctor before starting with a trainer.   Your doctor may want to refer you to a physical therapist before clearing you for exercise.   A physical therapist is a trained medical professional who will be able to incorporate all your medical issues into a specific exercise program designed for you.

TIPS FOR SETTING FITNESS GOALS

Start your exercise program by establishing fitness goals and develop a plan to achieve them.

1. Evaluate your current level of activity. You may be surprised at how much you move throughout the day.   A pedometer is an easy way to provide an initial assessment of your activity level.   Sportline is one of the recommended brands that you can purchase at a sporting goods store. Test the pedometer on a previously calculated path to ensure accuracy. After wearing a pedometer for a day or two, you can then set a goal to increase your activity to the next level to help you burn more calories.   A goal for most individuals is 10,000 steps daily, which roughly equals 5 miles.   The average person walks about 2-3 miles per day doing regular daily living activities.   Listed below is a chart with step goals per day:

STEPS/DAY	MILES WALKED/ DAY	LEVEL OF ACTIVITY
2,000	1.0	LOW
5,000	2.5	MEDIUM
10,000	5.0	OPTIMAL

2. **Short-term Goals.**   Start with short-term goals, such as biking for 20 minutes three times this week.   Achieving short-term goals will provide motivation to continue with a program.

3. **Start Slowly.**   Avoid an "all or nothing" mindset to prevent feelings of failure if you mess up.   Start slowly and build on your progress.   If you miss a workout, just pick up where you left off.

4. **Include Strength-Training.**   Try to include strength-training in your program.   Strength-training should ideally be done at least 2-3 times per week because it can prevent age-related loss of muscle mass and bone density.   In the long-run, it can help you move and function better.   For maximum effect, try moves that focus on big muscle groups like legs, butt, and back, such as "lunges," "squats," and "rows."

5. **Break exercise up throughout the day.**   Your exercise does not have to be all at one time.   Instead of trying to block off a 30-minute chunk of time in your schedule, block two 15-minute chunks of time to better fit exercise into your day.   Everything you do sums up to your total workout time.

TARGET HEART RATE

Although exercise can be broken up into 10-minute stints, it is important to note that you get the most out of your workout when your heart rate is at its target rate.   At your target heart rate, you are burning fat at the highest pace for your body.   In order to find your target heart rate, you need to first find your maximum heart rate.   This is calculated at 220 minus your age. Your target heart rate is between 50% and 75% of your maximum heart rate.   You can also use the table listed below as a short cut to finding your target heart rate based on your age.   It is recommended when beginning an exercise program to aim for the lower end of your target heart rate and gradually increase as weeks go on.

Calculate Your Target Heart Rate

Age	Target heart rate zone (50%-75%) beats per minute	Average maximum heart rate (100%) beats per minute
20	100-150	200
25	98-146	195
30	95-142	190
35	93-138	185
40	90-135	180
45	88-131	175
50	85-127	170
55	83-123	165
60	80-120	160
65	78-116	155
70	75-113	150

HURRY UP AND...WAIT

Do you ever find yourself rushing somewhere only to find that you must sit and wait?

These tips can increase your activity throughout the day

- Keep a pair of good walking shoes with you, in your desk or car, for unplanned exercise. Use a pedometer to measure the distance you've walked and the calories burned.

- Find a nearby area and go for a walk if you arrive too early. Waiting for your kids' baseball game to end? Athletic fields often have a walking path surrounding them and even office buildings may have long hallways that could serve as walking paths. Stairs can give you a workout that becomes cardiovascular if done for several minutes. If you spend a good deal of time in the car driving to appointments or picking up kids, try to arrive a few minutes early so you can take a brisk walk beforehand.

- If several of your appointments or pick-ups are in the same area, park the car and walk to each one. Park as far away as you can from an appointment to force yourself to walk further.

- Stuck waiting in the airport? Since new regulations recommend we arrive 2 hours before a flight, this is actually a great chance to get some walking done.

- Avoid the moving walkway at airports and get to your destination the old-fashioned way. Remember, extra minutes spent walking instead of sitting can make a difference in your weight and overall health.

It's a Date

Use your day planner to incorporate exercise into every day activities. At the beginning of each week, schedule time to exercise. In other words, make a "date" with yourself. However, it is important to be flexible in case something changes that forces you to miss your exercise date. Immediately reschedule any missed exercise to a better time, to better stay on track.

Here are some tips on how to maintain an exercise program

- **List Reasons for Exercise.** List the reasons why you have decided to regularly exercise on paper and put the list in a place you will see it every day, like the bathroom mirror, refrigerator, on your desk, or your car's dashboard. This will help reinforce exercise.

- **Find your Motivation by Asking a Friend.** Ask someone who exercises regularly why he does so. Find out what motivates him and how he works around his own schedule conflicts. Many busy people find ways to never miss their exercise.

- **Make Exercise a Routine Thing!** Think of exercise as part of your daily routine, just like taking a shower or brushing your teeth. The more you resist the temptation not to exercise, the less you'll feel that temptation and exercise will become a natural part of your daily routine.

- **Vary your exercise routine.** Avoid boredom by trying a new exercise before you have the chance to get bored with what you are doing.

- **Discover winter.** Winter can be a great time to exercise outdoors if you dress appropriately. Clear cold days and nights are perfect for a brisk walk or run. Take the dog or borrow a neighbor's. Better yet, volunteer at a shelter to walk dogs. You'll soon have a new buddy or two. Each season of the year has advantages, and seeing the different seasons on foot can be rewarding.

- **Vary Exercise Times.** Remember that exercise does not have to be done all at once. Try doing 15 minutes in the morning and another 15 minutes in the evening if that's what best fits your schedule.

- **Exercise with a friend.** This can be more fun and motivating. When you are both committed to a plan together, you can motivate each other and are less likely to skip a workout.

Chart Your Progress

An excellent way to keep your motivation is to keep an exercise log. In the log you record your workout goals and how you want to achieve them. Then you record exactly what you accomplished at each workout and the time you spent. A log can help track your progress and allow adjustments to your exercise routine as needed. As with a food log, an exercise log will hold you accountable for your fitness goals and keep you on track. It may also help you to identify situations that interfere with your goals.

FUELING FOR PERFORMANCE

For those that are already regularly exercising or training for an event, staying hydrated and fueled is crucial. Carbohydrates play a big role by fueling your muscles and brain. Dehydration (fluid loss) and hyponatremia (sodium loss) should also be a big concern. Hyponatremia can be caused by fluid loss or by drinking too much fluid before, during, or after the event. During training, find meals, snacks, and fluids that work best for you. Have your own personal recipe for fueling for success.

- Drink before you feel thirsty. Seniors and children tend to be less sensitive to the sensation of thirst. Besides water, sweat contains electrolytes that keep the fluid inside and outside of your cells in balance.

- Know your sweat rate. Begin by identifying your hourly fluid loss (especially when training for events) by weighing nude before and after a run and before eating and drinking. Any weight loss represents fluid loss, and you can base necessary fluid intake on this. A 2% loss in weight represents dehydration, and you can lose your ability to perform well. A 9 to 12% loss can cause death.

- Check your urine. Look for signs of dehydration. A light colored urine is well hydrated. A dark colored urine may indicate you need more fluids.

- Drink throughout the day. Prior to a long run (2 hours) , drink about 10 to 24 oz. of fluid and an additional 8 oz. 10 to 20 minutes before the run. Eat a few salty snacks to stimulate your thirst and help retain fluid.

- Avoid over hydrating. Drinking too much can lead to a dilution of your blood sodium resulting in hyponatremia.

- Drink sports drinks that contain about 14 to 19 grams of carbohydrate per 8 ounces. Higher concentrations of carbs can upset the stomach.

- Replace fluid and electrolyte losses. Drinking 50% more fluid than you lost in sweat will enhance recovery. If you become dehydrated drink frequently for the next day or two.

- Using sports drinks during exercise keeps you hydrated, maintains blood sugar, and adds important electrolytes (sodium and potassium).

- Eat high carbohydrate meals daily to fuel your muscles while training.

The night before an event eat a high carbohydrate meal and drink extra fluids.

- Start the day of an event with a combination of carbohydrates (bagel, banana) and protein (cheese or peanut butter).

- After an event remember to refuel muscle glycogen stores by eating carbohydrates within 30 minutes. Drink a sports drink and eat fruit or crackers. Use the formula about a half gram for every pound you weigh.

EXERCISE AND BUILDING STRONGER BONES

Getting adequate calcium and vitamin D are crucial to building strong bones. Numerous studies have found, however, that there is as strong a relationship between exercise and improvement in bone mineral density. These studies have shown that the pull of muscle on bone stimulates bone growth and allow bone to become stronger and denser. High impact exercise allows muscles and bones to work against gravity to build strength. Combining resistance and strength-training exercise helps to not only build bone but also builds muscle that supports the skeleton and improves balance and posture. This is crucial to preventing falls that lead to fractures. Dr. Miriam Nelson, director of Tufts University's John Hancock Research on Physical Activity, Nutrition, and Obesity Prevention recommends a program of exercise that combines aerobic, weight, and strength training. This allows maintaining fitness and bone density. Muscle strength and balance will aid in fall prevention. If you don't fall, you won't have to worry about a fracture.

With all these benefits, it's a wonder more Americans aren't exercising!

HIGH IMPACT EXERCISE	LOW IMPACT EXERCISE	NON-WEIGHT BEARING
• Dancing	• Elliptical training machine use	• Bicycling
• High impact aerobics		• Indoor cycling
• Hiking	• Fast walking on a treadmill or outside walking	• Deep-water walking
• Jogging or Running		• Flexibility exercise
• Jumping rope	• Low impact aerobics	• Stretching exercise
• Racket-ball	• Stair-step machine use	• Swimming
• Tennis		• Water aerobics
• Volleyball		

Check out www.bayerhearts.com for a 45 minute exercise program developed by the Bone Estrogen Strength Training Study (BEST) at University of Arizona. Videos are available to show how to properly perform the exercises. The National Osteoporosis Foundation at www.nof.org offers a similar program. The World Health Organization has developed a tool to assess fracture risk. You can find it at: http://www.shef.ac.uk/FRAX/tool.jsp?country=9

Below are a few exercise apps that you can use to help you reach your fitness goals:

1. Yoga with Janet Stone (iPhone, iPod touch, & iPad)
2. Endomondo Pro (Android, iPhone, & iPad)
3. Nike Training Club (Android, iPhone, iPod touch, & iPad)
4. Zombies, Run (iPhone, iPod touch, iPad, & coming to Android soon)

Answers to Exercise Questions

1. True

2. False--Americans should exercise for at least 30 minutes daily.

3. False-- Getting to and from a health club and or waiting to use equipment may take extra time.

4. True

5. True

6. False--an unwillingness to exercise will make it difficult to lose weight.

7. True

8. False--Carefully looking at your daily schedule will allow you to find ways to incorporate exercise.

Exercise Log for Week Ending _____

Day	Type of Exercise (weights, aerobic, other)	Duration	Intensity (minimal, challenging, strenuous)	Goal Accomplished (yes or no)	Notes
Sunday					
Monday					
Tuesday					
Wednesday					
Thursday					
Friday					
Saturday					

Activity, Exercise or Sport (1 hour)	130 lb	155 lb	180 lb	205 lb
Cycling, mountain bike, bmx	502	598	695	791
Cycling, <10 mph, leisure bicycling	236	281	327	372
Cycling, >20 mph, racing	944	1126	1308	1489
Cycling, 10-11.9 mph, light	354	422	490	558
Cycling, 12-13.9 mph, moderate	472	563	654	745
Cycling, 14-15.9 mph, vigorous	590	704	817	931
Cycling, 16-19 mph, very fast, racing	708	844	981	1117
Unicycling	295	352	409	465
Stationary cycling, very light	177	211	245	279
Stationary cycling, light	325	387	449	512
Stationary cycling, moderate	413	493	572	651
Stationary cycling, vigorous	620	739	858	977
Stationary cycling, very vigorous	738	880	1022	1163
Calisthenics, vigorous, pushups, situps...	472	563	654	745
Calisthenics, light	207	246	286	326
Circuit training, minimal rest	472	563	654	745
Weight lifting, body building, vigorous	354	422	490	558
Weight lifting, light workout	177	211	245	279
Health club exercise	325	387	449	512
Stair machine	531	633	735	838
Rowing machine, light	207	246	286	326
Rowing machine, moderate	413	493	572	651
Rowing machine, vigorous	502	598	695	791
Rowing machine, very vigorous	708	844	981	1117
Ski machine	413	493	572	651

Activity, Exercise or Sport (1 hour)	130 lb	155 lb	180 lb	205 lb
Aerobics, low impact	295	352	409	465
Aerobics, high impact	413	493	572	651
Aerobics, step aerobics	502	598	695	791
Aerobics, general	384	457	531	605
Jazzercise	354	422	490	558
Stretching, hatha yoga	236	281	327	372
Mild stretching	148	176	204	233
Instructing aerobic class	354	422	490	558
Water aerobics	236	281	327	372
Ballet, twist, jazz, tap	266	317	368	419
Ballroom dancing, slow	177	211	245	279
Ballroom dancing, fast	325	387	449	512
Running, 5 mph (12 minute mile)	472	563	654	745
Running, 5.2 mph (11.5 minute mile)	531	633	735	838
Running, 6 mph (10 min mile)	590	704	817	931
Running, 6.7 mph (9 min mile)	649	774	899	1024
Running, 7 mph (8.5 min mile)	679	809	940	1070
Running, 7.5mph (8 min mile)	738	880	1022	1163
Running, 8 mph (7.5 min mile)	797	950	1103	1256
Running, 8.6 mph (7 min mile)	826	985	1144	1303
Running, 9 mph (6.5 min mile)	885	1056	1226	1396
Running, 10 mph (6 min mile)	944	1126	1308	1489
Running, 10.9 mph (5.5 min mile)	1062	1267	1471	1675
Running, cross country	531	633	735	838

Activity, Exercise or Sport (1 hour)	130 lb	155 lb	180 lb	205 lb
Running, general	472	563	654	745
Running, on a track, team practice	590	704	817	931
Running, stairs, up	885	1056	1226	1396
Track and field (shot, discus)	236	281	327	372
Track and field (high jump, pole vault)	354	422	490	558
Track and field (hurdles)	590	704	817	931
Archery	207	246	286	326
Badminton	266	317	368	419
Basketball game, competitive	472	563	654	745
Playing basketball, non game	354	422	490	558
Basketball, officiating	413	493	572	651
Basketball, shooting baskets	266	317	368	419
Basketball, wheelchair	384	457	531	605
Running, training, pushing wheelchair	472	563	654	745
Billiards	148	176	204	233
Bowling	177	211	245	279
Boxing, in ring	708	844	981	1117
Boxing, punching bag	354	422	490	558
Boxing, sparring	531	633	735	838
Coaching: football, basketball, soccer…	236	281	327	372
Cricket (batting, bowling)	295	352	409	465
Croquet	148	176	204	233
Curling	236	281	327	372
Darts (wall or lawn)	148	176	204	233

Activity, Exercise or Sport (1 hour)	130 lb	155 lb	180 lb	205 lb
Fencing	354	422	490	558
Football, competitive	531	633	735	838
Football, touch, flag, general	472	563	654	745
Football or baseball, playing catch	148	176	204	233
Frisbee playing, general	177	211	245	279
Frisbee, ultimate frisbee	472	563	654	745
Golf, general	266	317	368	419
Golf, walking and carrying clubs	266	317	368	419
Golf, driving range	177	211	245	279
Golf, miniature golf	177	211	245	279
Golf, walking and pulling clubs	254	303	351	400
Golf, using power cart	207	246	286	326
Gymnastics	236	281	327	372
Hacky sack	236	281	327	372
Handball	708	844	981	1117
Handball, team	472	563	654	745
Hockey, field hockey	472	563	654	745
Hockey, ice hockey	472	563	654	745
Riding a horse, general	236	281	327	372
Horesback riding, saddling horse	207	246	286	326
Horseback riding, grooming horse	207	246	286	326
Horseback riding, trotting	384	457	531	605
Horseback riding, walking	148	176	204	233
Horse racing, galloping	472	563	654	745
Horse grooming, moderate	354	422	490	558

Activity, Exercise or Sport (1 hour)	130 lb	155 lb	180 lb	205 lb
Horseshoe pitching	177	211	245	279
Jai alai	708	844	981	1117
Martial arts, judo, karate, jujitsu	590	704	817	931
Martial arts, kick boxing	590	704	817	931
Martial arts, tae kwan do	590	704	817	931
Krav maga training	590	704	817	931
Juggling	236	281	327	372
Kickball	413	493	572	651
Lacrosse	472	563	654	745
Orienteering	531	633	735	838
Playing paddleball	354	422	490	558
Paddleball, competitive	590	704	817	931
Polo	472	563	654	745
Racquetball, competitive	590	704	817	931
Playing racquetball	413	493	572	651
Rock climbing, ascending rock	649	774	899	1024
Rock climbing, rappelling	472	563	654	745
Jumping rope, fast	708	844	981	1117
Jumping rope, moderate	590	704	817	931
Jumping rope, slow	472	563	654	745
Rugby	590	704	817	931
Shuffleboard, lawn bowling	177	211	245	279
Skateboarding	295	352	409	465
Roller skating	413	493	572	651
Roller blading, in-line skating	708	844	981	1117

Activity, Exercise or Sport (1 hour)	130 lb	155 lb	180 lb	205 lb
Sky diving	177	211	245	279
Soccer, competitive	590	704	817	931
Playing soccer	413	493	572	651
Softball or baseball	295	352	409	465
Softball, officiating	236	281	327	372
Softball, pitching	354	422	490	558
Squash	708	844	981	1117
Table tennis, ping pong	236	281	327	372
Tai chi	236	281	327	372
Playing tennis	413	493	572	651
Tennis, doubles	354	422	490	558
Tennis, singles	472	563	654	745
Trampoline	207	246	286	326
Volleyball, competitive	472	563	654	745
Playing volleyball	177	211	245	279
Volleyball, beach	472	563	654	745
Wrestling	354	422	490	558
Wallyball	413	493	572	651
Backpacking, Hiking with pack	413	493	572	651
Carrying infant, level ground	207	246	286	326
Carrying infant, upstairs	295	352	409	465
Carrying 16 to 24 lbs, upstairs	354	422	490	558
Carrying 25 to 49 lbs, upstairs	472	563	654	745
Standing, playing with children, light	165	197	229	261

Activity, Exercise or Sport (1 hour)	130 lb	155 lb	180 lb	205 lb
Walk/run, playing with children, moderate	236	281	327	372
Walk/run, playing with children, vigorous	295	352	409	465
Carrying small children	177	211	245	279
Loading, unloading car	177	211	245	279
Climbing hills, carrying up to 9 lbs	413	493	572	651
Climbing hills, carrying 10 to 20 lb	443	528	613	698
Climbing hills, carrying 21 to 42 lb	472	563	654	745
Climbing hills, carrying over 42 lb	531	633	735	838
Walking downstairs	177	211	245	279
Hiking, cross country	354	422	490	558
Bird watching	148	176	204	233
Marching, rapidly, military	384	457	531	605
Children's games, hopscotch, dodgeball	295	352	409	465
Pushing stroller or walking with children	148	176	204	233
Pushing a wheelchair	236	281	327	372
Race walking	384	457	531	605
Rock climbing, mountain climbing	472	563	654	745
Walking using crutches	295	352	409	465
Walking the dog	177	211	245	279
Walking, under 2.0 mph, very slow	118	141	163	186
Walking 2.0 mph, slow	148	176	204	233
Walking 2.5 mph	177	211	245	279
Walking 3.0 mph, moderate	195	232	270	307
Walking 3.5 mph, brisk pace	224	267	311	354

Activity, Exercise or Sport (1 hour)	130 lb	155 lb	180 lb	205 lb
Walking 3.5 mph, uphill	354	422	490	558
Walking 4.0 mph, very brisk	295	352	409	465
Walking 4.5 mph	372	443	515	586
Walking 5.0 mph	472	563	654	745
Boating, power, speed boat	148	176	204	233
Canoeing, camping trip	236	281	327	372
Canoeing, rowing, light	177	211	245	279
Canoeing, rowing, moderate	413	493	572	651
Canoeing, rowing, vigorous	708	844	981	1117
Crew, sculling, rowing, competition	708	844	981	1117
Kayaking	295	352	409	465
Paddle boat	236	281	327	372
Windsurfing, sailing	177	211	245	279
Sailing, competition	295	352	409	465
Sailing, yachting, ocean sailing	177	211	245	279
Skiing, water skiing	354	422	490	558
Ski mobiling	413	493	572	651
Skin diving, fast	944	1126	1308	1489
Skin diving, moderate	738	880	1022	1163
Skin diving, scuba diving	413	493	572	651
Snorkeling	295	352	409	465
Surfing, body surfing or board surfing	177	211	245	279
Whitewater rafting, kayaking, canoeing	295	352	409	465
Swimming laps, freestyle, fast	590	704	817	931
Swimming laps, freestyle, slow	413	493	572	651

Activity, Exercise or Sport (1 hour)	130 lb	155 lb	180 lb	205 lb
Swimming backstroke	413	493	572	651
Swimming breaststroke	590	704	817	931
Swimming butterfly	649	774	899	1024
Swimming leisurely, not laps	354	422	490	558
Swimming sidestroke	472	563	654	745
Swimming synchronized	472	563	654	745
Swimming, treading water, fast, vigorous	590	704	817	931
Swimming, treading water, moderate	236	281	327	372
Water aerobics, water calisthenics	236	281	327	372
Water polo	590	704	817	931
Water volleyball	177	211	245	279
Water jogging	472	563	654	745
Diving, springboard or platform	177	211	245	279
Ice skating, < 9 mph	325	387	449	512
Ice skating, average speed	413	493	572	651
Ice skating, rapidly	531	633	735	838
Speed skating, ice, competitive	885	1056	1226	1396
Cross country snow skiing, slow	413	493	572	651
Cross country skiing, moderate	472	563	654	745
Cross country skiing, vigorous	531	633	735	838
Cross country skiing, racing	826	985	1144	1303
Cross country skiing, uphill	974	1161	1348	1536
Snow skiing, downhill skiing, light	295	352	409	465

Activity, Exercise or Sport (1 hour)	130 lb	155 lb	180 lb	205 lb
Downhill snow skiing, moderate	354	422	490	558
Downhill snow skiing, racing	472	563	654	745
Sledding, tobagganing, luge	413	493	572	651
Snow shoeing	472	563	654	745
Snowmobiling	207	246	286	326
General housework	207	246	286	326
Cleaning gutters	295	352	409	465
Painting	266	317	368	419
Sit, playing with animals	148	176	204	233
Walk / run, playing with animals	236	281	327	372
Bathing dog	207	246	286	326
Mowing lawn, walk, power mower	325	387	449	512
Mowing lawn, riding mower	148	176	204	233
Walking, snow blower	207	246	286	326
Riding, snow blower	177	211	245	279
Shoveling snow by hand	354	422	490	558
Raking lawn	254	303	351	400
Gardening, general	236	281	327	372
Bagging grass, leaves	236	281	327	372
Watering lawn or garden	89	106	123	140
Weeding, cultivating garden	266	317	368	419
Carpentry, general	207	246	286	326
Carrying heavy loads	472	563	654	745
Carrying moderate loads upstairs	472	563	654	745

Activity, Exercise or Sport (1 hour)	130 lb	155 lb	180 lb	205 lb
General cleaning	207	246	286	326
Cleaning, dusting	148	176	204	233
Taking out trash	177	211	245	279
Walking, pushing a wheelchair	236	281	327	372
Teach physical education,exercise class	236	281	327	372
Teach exercise classes (& participate)	384	457	531	605

Source: NutriStrategy

SECTION 3

NUTRITION ISSUES INFLUENCING OUR HEALTH

CHOLESTEROL AND DIETARY FAT INTAKE

"HE WHO TAKES MEDICINE AND NEGLECTS TO DIET WASTES THE SKILL OF HIS DOCTORS." - CHINESE PROVERB

Check your understanding of Cholesterol by answering <u>True</u> or <u>False</u> to the following questions:

1. I should have my cholesterol checked yearly by my doctor.

2. My desirable total cholesterol should be less than 200 mg/dL.

3. There is no difference between HDL cholesterol and LDL cholesterol; they should both be low.

4. To lower my cholesterol, I only have to lower my dietary cholesterol intake.

5. The main source of dietary cholesterol comes from fruits and vegetables.

6. The majority of cholesterol in the body comes from the pancreas.

7. Palm oil and coconut oil are high in saturated fat.

The fast-paced lifestyles of today challenge even the most prudent dieter when it comes to trying to avoid high fat foods. Restaurant, carry-out, fast foods and grab-and-go foods can have more fat in a meal then one can imagine. In fact, unless you look at nutrition information (when available) and choose wisely, a single meal can provide an individual's daily quota of fat.

For years the quantity of fat as well as the type of fat that contributes to heart disease has been under debate and has been confusing. According to the USDA, Americans get about 35% of their total calories from solid fats and added sugars, and about 11 to 12% of calories from saturated fat. The new 2010 Dietary guidelines recommend reducing saturated fat to less than 7% of total calories and to replace saturated fat with monounsaturated and polyunsaturated fats. Avoid replacing fat with highly refined carbohydrates and added sugars. The guidelines also recommend shifting to a plant based diet by increasing intake of whole grains, vegetables, and fruits. Below we've provided you some of the key recommendations so you can achieve the health benefits of the new recommendations.

WHAT IS CHOLESTEROL?

Cholesterol is a soft fat-like substance that makes up part of our cells and tissues. It is part of a group of substances called *lipids*. During digestion of fat, cholesterol and fats are packaged (called a *lipoprotein*) in a certain way, enabling cholesterol to travel through the body. The liver makes some cholesterol naturally but the remainder of the cholesterol in your body comes from food sources. Since all animals naturally produce cholesterol, animal fat and skin are the main sources of cholesterol in the diet.

> **HDL carries cholesterol away from blood vessel walls to be excreted.**

There are 3 main types of lipoproteins you should be familiar with

- Very low-density lipoprotein (VLDL) cholesterol. VLDL carries fats to different parts of the body. VLDL is made in the liver and helps make LDL cholesterol.
- Low-density lipoprotein (LDL) cholesterol. LDL carries cholesterol to different parts of the body, and it is considered the "bad" cholesterol because it can stick to the inside of our blood vessels, making it harder for blood to pass through. This may increase your risk of heart disease.
- High density lipoprotein (HDL) cholesterol. This is known as the "good" cholesterol because HDL carries cholesterol away from blood vessel walls, carrying it back to the liver. The liver breaks down cholesterol to be excreted or recycled into new VLDL. Having more HDL and less LDL is beneficial.

Triglycerides are also a form of fat. These are part of lipoprotein particles found in the blood. Triglycerides are found in food and body fat. Your body stores the extra calories you eat as triglycerides. Having a high triglyceride level is often associated with a low HDL level, a combination associated with an increased risk of heart disease.

WHY DOES CHOLESTEROL MATTER?

Above normal cholesterol puts you at an increased risk for heart disease. Other factors include:

- Family history of heart disease
- Being 45 years or older for a man or 55 years or older for a woman
- Smoking
- High blood pressure
- Diabetes

When you eat excess fat in your diet, you can increase both your LDL levels and your risk of heart disease. The liver combines the fat and cholesterol from your diet into VLDL, which travels through your blood, unloading fat on its way. VLDL becomes LDL in the bloodstream and sticks to your blood vessel walls. The deposits of LDL cholesterol within the walls of the blood vessels are plaques and they narrow blood vessels and make them less flexible.

In a healthy person, HDL comes along and picks up LDL and returns it to the liver where it is either converted to new VLDL or broken down and excreted. Therefore, the ratio between total cholesterol and HDL cholesterol is a good predictor of heart disease because the more HDL and less LDL you have, the healthier your blood vessels will be.

One of the goals in managing cardiovascular disease is raising HDL cholesterol since HDL protects against heart disease. The National Cholesterol Education Program Adult Treatment Panel III recommends lifestyle changes as first-line treatment for increasing HDL cholesterol if levels are below 40 mg/dL. Exercise of moderate intensity more than three times per week will increase HDL cholesterol an average of 4%. A decrease of 1kg (2.2 lbs.) of body weight in overweight adults will increase HDL cholesterol by an average of 1%. Alcohol consumption of 1oz. may raise HDL cholesterol by 4 mg/dl, but this must be considered in light of potential risks of alcohol abuse and liver dysfunction. Stopping smoking may lead to a 3% to 5.6% increase in HDL cholesterol levels.

Target Levels for Blood Lipids	
Total Cholesterol	less than 200 mg/dL
LDL Cholesterol	less than 100 mg/dL
HDL Cholesterol	at least 40 mg/dL for men
	at least 50 mg/dL for women
Triglycerides	less than 150 mg/dL
Total Cholesterol:HDL Ratio	less than 3.0 mg/dL

Major risk factors that influence LDL cholesterol goals

- Cigarette smoking
- Hypertension (BP ≥ 140/90 or taking antihypertensive medication)
- Low HDL cholesterol (men <40 mg/dl, women <50 mg/dl)
- Family history of premature CHD (CHD in first degree male <55 yr/female <65 yr)
- Age (men ≥ 45 yr, women ≥ 55 yr)

THE TLC DIET

If you do have one or more of the major risk factors and your LDL level is greater than your goal, it is recommended you follow the TLC (Therapeutic Lifestyle Changes) diet.

TLC Diet Components

- **25-35% of total calories from fat**
    - Example: 1800 kcal diet = 540 calories, <60 grams fat per day
- **Less than 7% of total calories from saturated fat**
    - Example: 1800 calories x 7% = 126 calories, <14 grams sat fat per day
- **Less than 0.5% of total calories from Trans fat**
    - Example: 18 calories x 1% = 18 calories, <2 grams Trans fat per day
- **Less than 200 mg dietary cholesterol per day**
- **10-25 grams Soluble Fiber per day**
- **2 grams Plant Sterols/Stanols per day**

Following this diet, along with increased physical activity and weight management is a great start to lowering your LDL-cholesterol and thereby reducing your risk of developing heart disease.

CHOLESTEROL FROM FOOD

Cholesterol is not a nutritional necessity in the diet, because our bodies make enough to live and perform properly. Therefore, it would be wise to eat foods naturally low in cholesterol or, preferably, cholesterol-free.

Avoiding high fat, high cholesterol foods can be tricky especially for the busy person. Carry-out or convenience foods are usually loaded with fat, which raises cholesterol. Restaurant foods are often cooked with more fat than necessary and the portion size of meat is usually much larger than needed. Know your cuts of meat and choose wisely. Avoiding a high fat, high cholesterol diet takes knowledge and planning. A good start is to assess your current fat intake. New restaurant legislation passed in 2010 will make eating out easier. Restaurants and vendors with more than 20 locations will have to disclose calorie and other nutrient information. You can also estimate the amount of fat in restaurant foods by using charts found at www.CalorieKing.com, or purchase the pocket sized book at your local bookstore.

What you can do if your blood lipids are above recommended levels	
• Work with a dietitian to develop an individualized meal plan	• Choose whole-grain breads and cereals
• Use less oil, butter, margarine, and other fats	• Try to exercise for 30 minutes most days
• Choose low-fat dairy instead of full-fat	• Know your medications and their interactions
• Eat smaller servings of meat, fish, and poultry	• Quit smoking
• Eat more fresh fruits and vegetables	• Use food products that contain plant sterols
• Maintain a healthy weight	• Include unsalted tree nuts (almonds, walnuts, pistachios), peanuts, and seeds
	• 8-12 oz. per week of seafood high in omega-3, e.g., salmon

Following this diet, along with increased physical activity and weight management, is a great start to lowering your LDL-cholesterol and thereby reducing your risk of developing heart disease.

TYPES OF FAT

Studies have shown that with an increase in trans fat there is an increase in cardiovascular disease. In fact, a study from 2006 in The New England Journal of Medicine showed a 23% increase risk for heart disease with approximately 4 grams of trans fats in a 2,000 calorie diet. Denmark passed legislation which almost eliminates the use of trans fats, resulting in about 60% decline in cardiovascular disease. Currently there is no recommended safe level for trans fatty acids in the diet. The American Heart Association recommends limiting trans fats to 2 g based on a 2,000 calorie diet.

Trans fats are now required to be listed on food labels. Since the FDA allows products with <0.5 g trans fat to claim 0 grams trans fats the labeling may be misleading; and consumers may be taking in more than they realize. As an example, if you have four servings of this food in one day, you have taken in 2 grams of trans fat, and that could push you over the recommended intake. Check the nutrition label. If the words *hydrogenation* or *partial hydrogenation* appear, you should count that food as having at least 0.5 grams trans fat.

Although many companies are eliminating trans fats from their food, they are often adding saturated fat, which is just as detrimental to the body. Interestingly, both trans and saturated fats raise LDL (bad cholesterol) and lower HDL (good cholesterol). Therefore, it is strongly recommended to avoid trans fat and saturated fat to avoid the associated health problems.

Trans Fats and Hydrogenation

Defined: Currently there is no recommended safe level for trans fatty acids in the diet. Though some trans fats occur naturally in foods, most are the result of adding hydrogen to liquid oil. This chemical change hardens the oil, a process called hydrogenation. Hydrogenation causes these oils to become similar to saturated fats and lengthens the shelf-life of food products. However, research shows that eating foods with hydrogenated oils increase the risk of heart disease.

Affect on Cholesterol: Trans fats and hydrogenated fats can increase LDL cholesterol and triglycerides and decrease HDL cholesterol, the "good" cholesterol.

Food Sources of Trans fat:
- Vegetable shortening
- Some margarines
- Commercially prepared foods and fried foods like:
  - Potato chips
  - Crackers
  - Cookies
  - Cakes

Saturated Fats

Defined: Generally, saturated fats are solid at room temperature. You can find the grams of saturated fat on packaged food labels.

Affect on Cholesterol: This fat is the biggest dietary contributor to heart disease because it tends to raise LDL cholesterol levels and lower HDL cholesterol.

Food Sources of Saturated Fat:

- Meat
- Cheese
- Butter
- Lard
- Eggs
- Dairy products
- Palm oil and coconut oil
- Most processed foods

Foods High in Saturated Fat and Cholesterol	
Meats	Some cuts of beef, pork, lamb products
	Regular ground beef (choose 90% lean)
	Spare ribs
	Organ meats – liver, kidneys
	Poultry with skin
	Fried chicken, fried fish, and fried shellfish
	Bologna, salami, sausage, and hot dogs
	All visible fat on meat is saturated, trim all visible fat from meats
	All visible skin, chicken and poultry, is saturated. Trim all skin from meats.
	Not all red meats are high in fat. In fact, many red meats are lean and can be worked into your diet. Check out the list of lean meat choices at the end of this chapter.
Eggs	1 egg has about 250 mg cholesterol, found in the yolk.
	It is recommended to eat no more than 2-3 egg yolks per week.
Dairy Products	Milk (both whole and 2%) – choose low fat varieties
	Whole milk yogurt and yogurt beverages - Choose low fat varieties
	Regular cheese look for part skim or skim, for example mozzarella and ricotta
	Cream, half and half, whipping cream, and nondairy creamer - low fat varieties
	Whipped topping
	Sour cream – choose low-fat, fat-free, or just skip it if only a condiment
Fats and Oils	Coconut oil
	Palm kernel oil
	Butter and margarine
	Lard
	Bacon fat
	Salad dressings
Fried Foods	Anything deep-fried, such as fried chicken, French fries, tortilla chips
Creamed Foods	Creamy sauces, gravies, and soups
	Substitute lower fat ingredients when preparing these foods at home
Commercially Prepared Baked Foods and Desserts	Many of these foods are made from the bad kind of fats like palm oil or coconut oil. These oils are less expensive for manufactures to use and are therefore often found in baked goods. Make your own dessert or enjoy some fruit at the end of the meal.

Comparison of Saturated Fat in Lean Meat Choices

Lean Red Meat Cuts:	Calories	Saturated Fat (g)	Total Fat (g)
Eye Round Roast and Steak*	144	1.4	4.0
Sirloin Tip Side Steak	143	1.6	4.1
Top Round Roast and Steak*	157	1.6	4.6
Bottom Round Roast and Steak*	139	1.7	4.9
Top Sirloin Steak	156	1.9	4.9
Brisket, Flat Half	167	1.9	5.1
95% Lean Ground Beef	139	2.3	5.1
Round Tip Roast and Steak*	148	1.9	5.3
Round Steak	154	1.9	5.3
Shank Cross Cuts	171	1.9	5.4
Chuck Shoulder Pot Roast	147	1.8	5.7
Sirloin Tip Center Roast and Steak*	150	2.1	5.8
Chuck Shoulder Steak	161	1.9	6.0
Bottom Round (Western Griller) Steak	155	2.2	6.0
Top Loin (Strip) Steak	161	2.6	6.0
Shoulder Petite Tender and Medallions*	150	2.4	6.1
Flank Steak	158	2.6	6.3
Shoulder Center (Ranch) Steak	155	2.4	6.5
Tri-Tip Roast and Steak*	158	2.6	7.1
Tenderloin Roast and Steak*	170	2.7	7.1
T-Bone Steak	172	3.0	8.2
Lean White Meat Cuts:[1]			
Pork Tenderloin, separated lean white meat only	104	1.0	2.8
Skinless Chicken Thigh	188	2.7	9.8
Skinless Chicken Breast	148	0.9	3.2
White Tuna Canned in Water	109	0.7	2.5
Salmon	175	2.1	10.5

Calories and fat based on 3-ounce servings, visible fat trimmed, and then 95 milligrams of cholesterol per 3-ounce serving.

*Cuts combined for illustration purposes.

Source: U.S. Department of Agriculture, Agricultural Research Service, 2008. USDA Nutrient Database for Standard Reference, Release 21.

[1]Source: U.S. Department of Agriculture, Agricultural Research Service, 2009. USDA Nutrient Database for Standard Reference, Release 22.

Monounsaturated Fats

Defined: Monounsaturated fats are liquid at room temperature but become solid when refrigerated. Try to shift to using these types of fats when preparing and choosing your foods.

Affect on Cholesterol: Monounsaturated fats actually seem to reduce LDL cholesterol and total cholesterol and keep HDL the same, which is good news.

Food Sources of Monounsaturated Fat:
- Canola oil
- Olive oil
- Almond and peanut oils
- Almonds*
- Avocados
- Peanut Oil
- Sunflower Oil
- Sesame oil
- Peanut Butter

*Almonds are also an excellent source of the antioxidant alpha-tocopherol from Vitamin E. This antioxidant has been shown to prevent cholesterol from sticking to artery walls. One ounce of almonds (about 23 almonds) has 160 calories and 7.4 mg of alpha-tocopherol. That is about half the calories of 2 ounces of potato chips or a candy bar, making almonds and other nuts a good snack choice.

Polyunsaturated Fats

Defined: Polyunsaturated fats are also liquid at room temperature, but unlike monounsaturated fats, these remain liquid even when refrigerated. Polyunsaturated fats are probably the most commonly used fats in the family kitchen.

Affect on Cholesterol: Polyunsaturated fats are known to lower LDL cholesterol, which is good, but it also lowers HDL cholesterol, which is not so good.

Food Sources of Polyunsaturated Fat:
- Corn oil
- Soybean oil
- Safflower oil
- Sunflower oil
- Walnuts - have also been shown in studies to reduce cholesterol and LDL levels.
- Margarine - yet if eaten in large quantities may also have a negative effect by reducing HDL

Omega-3 Fatty Acids

Defined: These are a type of polyunsaturated fat that also provide protection against heart disease. There are three types of omega-3 fatty acids: alpha-linolenic acid (ALA), eicosapentaenoic acid (EPA), and docosahexanoic acid (DHA). The body uses EPA and DHA more efficiently, whereas ALA requires further conversion.

Affect on Cholesterol: Omega-3 fatty acids can aid in reducing the risk of heart disease by making the blood less "sticky" and less likely to clot. They can also lower triglycerides. For heart protection, the recommendation for omega-3 fatty acids per day is 1 gram. However, for lowering triglycerides, 2 to 4 grams per day have been shown to be beneficial.

Food Sources of Omega-3 Fatty Acids:
- Fatty fish like salmon, mackerel, herring, and sardines - at least 2 servings of fatty fish per week are recommended
- Walnuts
- Flaxseed
- Canola oil
- Soy

Phytosterols

Defined: Phytosterols are also known as plant sterols. These cholesterol-like substances naturally occur in plants such as grains, nuts and legumes, vegetable oils, vegetables, and fruits. Though similar in structure to animal cholesterol, phytosterols actually help lower blood cholesterol levels. At the end of this chapter there are two charts which can help you identify what products contain plant sterols.

Affect on Cholesterol: They slow or prevent the absorption of cholesterol from your food and the cholesterol produced by the liver, preventing cholesterol from entering your blood. Although many foods on the market contain phytosterols, long-term studies are not available yet to know their long-term effects.

Food Products containing Phytosterols:
- Promise Activ Spread
- Take Control
- Benecol
- Smart Balance
- Health Valley Heart Wise Cereal and Granola Bars
- Minute Maid Premium Heart Wise Orange Juice
- Kroger Active Lifestyle Fat Free Milk

The product CholestOff by Nature Made blends plant sterols and stanols inhibiting the absorption of cholesterol from food causing some of it to pass through the body.

Table 1. Plant Sterols in Edible Oils and Foods *(in mg of plant sterols per unit of fresh food)*

Food Item	Total Plant Sterols
OILS (1tbsp)	
CORN OIL	100.0-133.3
COTTONSEED OIL	24.0-29.2
OLIVE OIL (EXTRA VIRGIN)	10.7-11.1
PALM OIL	3.6-4.5
RAPSEED OIL	35.0-102.0
CANOLA OIL	89.1-91.3
RICE BRAN OIL	77.6
SOYBEAN OIL	30.1-44.7
SUNFLOWER OIL	27.5-53.3
CEREAL GRAINS (.25 CUP)	
RYE	38.4-46.5
WHEAT	28.9-33.1
OATS	12.8-20.3
BARLEY	29.3-41.5
VEGETABLES (1 CUP)	
CORN	274.1
BRUSSEL SPROUTS	37.8
BROCCOLI	35.5
CAULIFLOWER	40.0
CARROT	20.5
POTATO	14.0
APPLE	16.3
ORANGE	43.2
LEGUMES (.75CUP)	
CHICKPEA	174.8-188.9
LENTIL	160.8-177.0
WHITE BEAN	155.0-172.6
PEANUT	52.3-55.4

Table 1. Plant Sterols in Edible Oils and Foods Continued *(in mg of plant sterols per unit of fresh food)*

Food Item	Total Plant Sterols
NUTS AND SEEDS	
ALMOND	25.2-26.8
HAZELNUT	23.0-24.5
PISTACHIO	48.2-50.5
SUNFLOWER SEED	39.3-41.7
WALNUT	16.0-16.8

Published with permission from the Diabetes Care and Education Dietetic Practice Group of the Academy of Nutrition and Dietetics:
Rideout TC, Lun B. Plant Sterols in the Management of Dyslipidemia in Patients with Diabetes. *On the Cutting Edge*. 2010;31(6):13-17.

Table 2. Selected Commercially Available Plant Sterol (PS)–Fortified Products

Brand	Product Name	Plant Sterol Content
SPREADS		
BENECOL	REGULAR & LIGHT SPREADS	850 mg/tbsp
TAKE CONTROL	PROMISE ACTIVE SPREADS (BUTTERY & LIGHT)	1,000 mg/tbsp
BEVERAGES		
MINUTE MAID	HEART WISE ORANGE JUICE	1,000 mg/8 fluid ounces
MILKS		
RICE DREAM	HEARTWISE (ORIGINAL & VANILLA)	650 mg/8 fluid ounces
SILK	HEART HEALTH SOY MILK	650 mg/8 fluid ounces
GIANT EAGLE	FAT FREE MILK	400mg/8 fluid ounces
KROGER	ACTIVE LIFESTYLE FAT-FREE MILK	400mg/8 fluid ounces
CHEESE		
LIFELINE	LIFETIME LOW FAT CHEESE (CHEDDAR, MOZZARELLA, SWISS, JALAPEÑO JACK, ETC.)	650mg/ounce
CHEWS		
QUEST	CARDIO CHEWS (CHEWY, CHOCOLATE)	400mg/chew
BENECOL	SMART CHEWS	850 mg/chew

Table 2. Commercially Available Plant Sterol-Fortified Products Continued

Brand	Product Name	Plant Sterol Content
BAKED GOODS		
KROGER	ACTIVE LIFESTYLE BREAD	800mg/serving
KRUSTEAZ	HEALTHY START PANCAKES AND WAFFLES	650mg/serving
VITAMUFFIN	DARK CHOCOLATE POMEGRANATE VITATOPS	400mg/top
PASTAS		
RACCONTO	HEART HEALTH PASTAS	400mg/serving

Published with permission from the Diabetes Care and Education Dietetic Practice Group of the Academy of Nutrition and Dietetics:
Rideout TC, Lun B. Plant Sterols in the Management of Dyslipidemia in Patients with Diabetes. *On the Cutting Edge*. 2010;31 (6):13-17.

KNOW YOUR OILS

In addition to nutrition, choose oils for flavor and consider their cooking characteristics. The smoke point refers to the temperature at which cooking oil breaks down and will begin to smoke or flame, and both flavor and nutrition are altered at this point. Another concern is that high cooking temperatures of unsaturated oils can convert them to saturated oils. For this reason, deep frying is not recommended.

The Low Down on Oils

- **Extra virgin olive oil:** Contains mostly monounsaturated fat. It has a light, peppery flavor and low smoke point. The low smoke point makes this oil better for a quick sauté of fish or other meats, and even better as a dressing for topping off salads and vegetables.
- **Olive oil:** Good for sautéing or adding to salads, vegetables.
- **Canola oil:** Contains mostly monounsaturated fat with the least amount of saturated fat of the oils. It has a neutral flavor and high smoke point making it good for frying and baking.
- **Peanut oil:** Contains about 50 percent monounsaturated fat and about 30 percent polyunsaturated fat. This oil is good for light sautéing.
- **Corn oil/vegetable oil:** High in polyunsaturated fat it has a high smoke point which makes this oil good for frying.
- **Sunflower and safflower oil:** High in polyunsaturated fat and it is good for high heat cooking
- **Flaxseed oil:** Best used for salad dressings

Fish is a great source of protein and is low in calories and saturated fat. It is also high in the omega-3 fats EPA and DHA. Some fish though contain mercury and persistent organic pollutants (POP). The 2010 Dietary Guidelines recommend 8 to 12 ounces of seafood per week for Americans. The Food and Drug Administration (FDA) and the Environmental Protection Agency (EPA) advise women who may become pregnant, pregnant women, nursing mothers, and young children to avoid the types of fish that are higher in mercury. Following is a list of fish and their mercury content.

AVOID	Omega-3 fatty acids (grams per 3-oz.)	Mean mercury level in parts per million (ppm)
Swordfish	0.97	0.97
Shark	0.83	0.99
King mackerel	0.36	0.73
Tilefish (golden bass or golden snapper)	0.90	1.45

Top 10 Fish Based on Omega-3 and Mercury Levels		
	Omega-3 fatty acids (grams per 3-oz.)	Mean mercury level in parts per million (ppm)
Canned tuna (light)	0.17-0.24	0.12
Shrimp	0.29	Below detection levels
Pollock	0.45	0.06
Salmon (fresh, frozen)	1.1-1.9	0.01
Cod	0.15-0.24	0.11
Catfish	0.22-0.3	0.05
Clams	0.25	Below detection levels
Flounder or sole	0.48	0.05
Crabs	0.27-0.40	0.06
Scallops	0.18-0.34	0.05

*** Source for above tables: Natural Resource Defense Council, adapted from FDA guidelines ***

Albacore ("white") tuna has more mercury than canned light tuna. So, when chosing your two meals of fish and shellfish, you may eat up to 6 ounces (one average meal) of albacore tuna per week.

NUTTY NUTRITION

Tree nuts provide an abundance of nutrition. They are rich in protein, minerals, fiber, phytonutrients, antioxidants, vitamin E, manganese, thiamin, phosphorus, and magnesium.

Tree Nut (raw)	Saturated Fat (g)
Almonds	1
Brazils	4
Cashews	2
Hazelnuts	1
Macadamias	3
Pecans	2
Pine Nuts	1
Pistachios	2
Walnuts	2

©2012, *Weight Management Matters* Newsletter; Weight Management, a dietetic practice group of the Academy of Nutrition and Dietetics. Used with permission

Answers to Cholesterol Questions
1. True
2. True
3. False. HDL is the "good" cholesterol that protects against heart disease. High levels are desirable.
4. False. You should lower the total amount of fat in your diet and thus lower the amount of saturated fat consumed.
5. False. Dietary cholesterol is found in animal foods. Fruits and vegetables contain no cholesterol.
6. False. Cholesterol is formed in the liver.
7. True

SODIUM

"CAN THAT WHICH IS UNSAVORY BE EATEN WITHOUT SALT?" - JOB 6:61

Sodium Questions: Answer <u>True</u> or <u>False</u> to the following questions concerning sodium in your diet.

1. The amount of sodium I eat is only a concern if I have high blood pressure in my family's disease history.
2. We should try to consume less than 2,400 mg of sodium a day.
3. A teaspoon of salt contains approximately 3000 mg of sodium.
4. Most dietary sodium comes from processed foods.
5. A high sodium intake places an individual at risk for hypertension and heart disease.

It's hard to imagine a meal without a bit of salt. Salt enhances the flavor of food, and without it many foods are bland and tasteless. For some, salt may be an acquired taste, and many people have become accustomed to eating more than what is necessary. Eating fresh, unprocessed foods is the easiest way to avoid taking in large amounts of sodium. Eating healthy includes taking a look at the amount of salt you use daily. Are you guilty of salting before tasting your food?

It may seem impossible to avoid sodium. Most foods contain some natural sodium. Prepared foods contain added sodium, and then there's the sodium we add to food while cooking and eating. Here's the breakdown on sources of sodium in our diet:

- 5% added during cooking
- 6% added during eating
- 12% found naturally in foods
- 77% found in prepared and processed food

Why do you need sodium?

....

- Sodium maintains the balance of fluids in the body
- Sodium transmits nerve impulses
- Sodium helps with contraction and relaxation of muscles

HOW MUCH IS ENOUGH?

Recently the spotlight has been on salt and its role in the American diet. The average American's intake is as much as 5,000 mg a day, and yet The National Academy of Science's Institute of Medicine states that 1500 mg of sodium per day is adequate for good health. The new 2010 Dietary Guidelines recommend limiting salt intake to 2,300 mg a day: about 1 teaspoon of salt. Some individuals are considered "salt sensitive". This includes individuals older than 51, African Americans, those with high blood pressure, or those with a family history of high BP. They may need to reduce their salt intake to 1,500 mg a day, about 2/3 teaspoon of salt.

Some experts link high sodium intake to hypertension, cardiovascular disease, kidney disease, and stroke. Yet there are some who disagree. The Salt Institute says the initiative to reduce sodium is "not based on sound science" pointing out that Italians, as well as people who make up the Mediterranean regions, use quite a bit of salt. They salt their fresh vegetables, fish, and meat and use it to age and dry-cure meats. And yet they have much lower incidence of cardiovascular disease.

What's one to believe? Is it the wrong kind of fat and calories, not to mention the added chemicals in highly processed foods, that make Americans unhealthy or is sodium to blame?

The Dietary Approaches to Stop Hypertension Study (DASH) found that blood pressure was lowered in the participants who reduced their sodium intake to 1,500 mg per day. Other studies have suggested a link between sodium and stomach cancer and the worsening of asthma. Sodium can also increase the excretion of calcium into the urine which may increase bone loss and the risk of kidney stones.

So, as the sodium debate continues we'll recommend that you continue to find ways to eat more fresh and unprocessed food—discovering along the way the variety of herbs and spices that can add flavor to foods—and use salt in moderation.

BECOME A SODIUM SLEUTH

The biggest contributor to sodium in the diet is from restaurant and processed foods. If you eat out frequently the likelihood is high that you are getting too much sodium. Here are a few examples of how much sodium is in restaurant foods. A Mc Donald's Sausage and Biscuit with Egg has 1,280 mg of sodium. A bowl of Broccoli Cheddar soup from Panera has 1,000 mg of sodium, and Olive Garden Chicken Parmigiana and Spaghetti has 3,380 mg. Who would have thought that the Garden Fare: Capellini de Mare (dinner portion) would contain 1,830mg sodium?

In April 2010, the FDA announced it will seek cooperation with the food industry to voluntarily reduce the salt in food and beverages. Reading food labels is essential to avoid foods containing large amounts of sodium. Packaged and processed foods are usually loaded with sodium, since salt is used to flavor and preserve these foods. These foods contribute the most sodium to the American diet. Look for foods labeled "reduced sodium".

The Percent Daily Value allows you to compare different products and details the amount of sodium (5% DV or less is low; 20% DV or more is high), telling you if a food is high or low in sodium. Labels provide the sodium content in milligrams for a single serving. The Percent (%) Daily Values on a label indicate how much of a nutrient one serving of food contains compared to recommendations for an entire day. The percent is based on a 2,000-calorie diet. The Daily Values would differ for individuals whose calorie intake is less or more than a 2,000-calorie diet.

LABEL LINGO

Know that there are certain terms that can only be used when the sodium level in the food item meets a defined level. Opt for "low-sodium" products. Their availability has more than doubled in the past 5 years.

Salt Free (or Sodium Fee)	Less than 5 mg sodium per serving
No Salt added	No salt added during processing; but does not mean sodium free
Very Low Sodium	35 mg or less sodium per serving
Low Sodium	140 mg or less per serving
Light in Sodium	50% less sodium (as compared with a standard serving size of the traditional food), restricted to those foods that have more than 40 calories per serving or more than 3 grams of fat per serving
Less Sodium or Reduced Sodium	Minimum of 25% less sodium (as compared to a standard serving size of the traditional food). These foods may still have a significant amount of sodium.

Some over-the-counter drugs contain sodium. Be sure to read the label before taking drugs, such as antacids. If an antacid contains 5 mg or more of sodium per serving, it must be listed on the label. Watch out for the word "soda," referring to sodium bicarbonate or baking soda. These products are made up of sodium compounds.

REDUCING YOUR SODIUM

Your goal is to stay within the recommended 2,300 mg of sodium daily. Balancing a high sodium meal with a meal that is fresh and unprocessed will help you stay within that daily sodium intake limit. Lowering salt intake doesn't mean you have to forfeit flavor. Follow these tips to help with ordering in a restaurant. Start with small lifestyle changes, and work up to larger dietary changes.

When adding sodium to foods, either using a salt shaker or when cooking, these quantities can give you an idea of the sodium content for each serving:

¼ teaspoon salt contains	=	575 mg sodium
½ teaspoon salt contains	=	1,150 mg sodium
¾ teaspoon salt contains	=	1,725 mg sodium
1 teaspoon salt contains	=	2,300 mg sodium
1 teaspoon baking soda	=	1,000 mg sodium

Tips for Reducing Sodium in Your Diet

1. Buy fresh or frozen vegetables. If you buy canned vegetables, look for items without added salt or rinse the vegetables in water before cooking.
2. Limit processed foods by limiting the use of canned, cured, processed or smoked meats and packaged and convenience foods.
3. Limit foods that are packed in brine: e.g., pickles, olives, sauerkraut, pickled vegetables.
4. Limit condiments that are high in sodium: e.g., soy sauce, garlic salt, bouillon cubes, Worcestershire sauce. Instead, use spices and herbs to enhance flavor.
5. Limit the number of salty snacks. These include: chips, pretzels, and snack crackers. You can also get many of these items without salt. Choose unsalted nuts and seeds.
6. Limit the use of fast foods. Check the nutrition content of fast foods. Most often, any one item will exceed the daily requirement for sodium.
7. Cook without using salt. Cook rice, pasta, and hot cereals without salt.
8. Read labels for sodium content. Food labels identify sodium in milligrams per serving. Keep an eye on the number of servings you would consume to determine if the product is safe for you to consume.

Lifestyle Changes, Starting Gradually

1. Remove the salt shaker from the table. Gradually reduce your salt intake. You'll enjoy the natural flavor of foods.
2. Spice up your life. Try using a variety of spices and herbs to enhance the taste of foods.
3. Herbs instead of salt. Fresh herbs combined enhance the flavor of food.
4. Restaurant Ordering Techniques. If you decide to reduce your salt intake and dine out frequently you will need to order smart. Brush up on restaurant ordering techniques. Go online and see how much sodium is in your favorite fast-food restaurant's fare.

Spices, flavorings, vegetables, and herbs can be used to naturally enhance the flavors of food. Sea salt and kosher salt still contain the same amount of

Restaurant Choices for Reducing Sodium

1. **Sauces:** Limit foods with sauces.
2. **Breaded and Fried:** Avoid breaded and fried foods as these can be high in sodium. Instead, ask for baked or broiled meats and fish when eating out.
3. **Marinated:** Limit marinated meats due to the high sodium content of these products.
4. **Start the meal with Vegetables or Fruit.** Soups are usually high in sodium; choose a salad or fresh fruit instead.
5. **Food Preparation Techniques:** Ask the waiter if the dishes can be prepared without added salt. Select foods prepared with healthy techniques such as steamed, grilled, broiled, baked, roasted, poached, or stir-fried.
6. **Ethnic Dishes:** Chinese, Japanese, Mexican, and Indian foods tend to be very high in sodium.
7. **Salad Dressing:** Use lemon juice or dressings on the side to enhance flavor of salads.
8. **Condiments:** Choose fresh tomato, lettuce, and cucumber accompaniments for sandwiches rather than olives, pickles, or sauces. Go easy on condiments; ketchup, sauces, cheese, and mayonnaise are hidden sources of sodium.

sodium by weight, but often are move flavorful. Experiment by utilizing the following guide, and find the combinations you prefer. Two websites that you can check for more info are: www.spiceadvice.com and www.nhlbi.nih.gov/hbp/prevent/sodium/flavor.htm.

Replace Salt with Herbs and Spices	
Beef	Allspice, bay leaf, caraway seeds, curry powder, dill, dry mustard, ginger, mushrooms, onions, onion flakes, pepper, sage, thyme, and tomatoes
Fish	Allspice, curry powder, Dijon mustard, dill, ginger, green pepper, honey, mushrooms, mustard, lemon, lemon pepper, tarragon, thyme, and tomatoes
Lamb	Curry powder, dill, mint, and sage
Pork	Basil, caraway, Dijon mustard, dry mustard, honey mustard, nutmeg, rosemary, and tarragon
Poultry	Bay leaf, dill, curry powder, ginger, green pepper, lemon, lemon pepper, marjoram, mushrooms, poultry seasoning, rosemary, sage, tarragon, thyme, and tomatoes
Veal	Bay leaf, curry powder, mushrooms, mustard, tarragon, and tomatoes

Replace Salt with Herbs and Spices Continued	
Chicken	Ginger, marjoram, oregano, paprika, rosemary, sage, tarragon, and thyme
Carrots	Cinnamon, cloves, marjoram, nutmeg, rosemary, and sage
Corn	Cumin, curry powder, onion, paprika, and parsley
Green Beans	Dill, curry powder, lemon juice, marjoram, oregano, tarragon, and thyme
Greens	Onion and pepper
Peas	Ginger, marjoram, onion, parsley, and sage
Potatoes	Dill, garlic, onion, paprika, parsley, and sage
Summer Squash	Cloves, curry powder, marjoram, nutmeg, rosemary, and sage
Winter Squash	Cinnamon, ginger, nutmeg, and onion
Tomatoes	Basil, bay leaf, dill, marjoram, onion, oregano, parsley, and pepper

Types of Salt	
Table Salts	Salt (plain & iodized)
Reduced Sodium Products	Salt substitute is 100% potassium chloride
	Morton Lite Salt Mixture is 50% sodium chloride (NaCl) and 50% potassium chloride (KCl)
	Morton Salt Balance Salt Blend is 75% NaCl and 25% KCl
	Salt Sense is 100% sodium. The salt crystal is puffed making it bigger than a normal crystal. There is 33% less salt in the container.
Gourmet and Specialty Salts	Coarse Kosher Salt
	Sea Salt (Fine & Coarse)
	Popcorn Salt
	Canning & Pickling Salt
	Ice Cream Salt

Types of Salt Continued		
Seasoned & Flavored Salts	Morton's Nature's Seasons Seasoning Blend	
	Garlic Salt	
	Seasoned Salt	
	Hot Salt	
	Sausage & Meat Loaf Seasoning Mix	

Potassium is the mineral substituted for sodium in salt substitutes. It has an unpleasant metallic aftertaste. By cooking with extra spices you can mask some of this flavor. Morton Salt Balance Salt Blend is only 25% potassium chloride (KCl). You get a 25% reduction in sodium and can't taste the KCl.

Remember that sodium is an essential nutrient to life and good health. However, it is important to be aware of the amount of sodium you take in since moderate salt intake is part of a healthy diet and lifestyle. So... Are you salting before tasting?

Answers to the Sodium Questions

1. False. As sodium intake increases so does blood pressure.
2. False. The daily sodium recommendation is less than 2,300 mg per day.
3. False. One teaspoon of salt contains 2,400 mg of sodium.
4. True
5. True

FIBER

Fiber Questions: Test your knowledge of dietary fiber consumption by answering <u>True</u> or <u>False</u> to the questions below.

1. The average American consumes only 10-15 grams of fiber daily.

2. Fiber should be added gradually to the diet along with plenty of fluids.

3. Some individuals may experience side effects when adding high fiber foods to their diet.

4. Eating high fiber foods will cause weight gain.

5. Women should eat 15 grams of fiber daily and men 20 grams.

We often turn our noses up at the thought of high fiber foods.   Yet many high fiber foods taste good, fit easily into a daily meal plan, and make us feel full between meals.   Eating high fiber foods is part of a healthy diet. Although this is yet one more thing to consider with a busy schedule, it is one we can't afford to ignore.

Despite research demonstrating the many health benefits of a high fiber and whole grain diet, America's intake is quite low. The average American consumes 1 or fewer servings of whole grains, which is less than 15 grams of fiber a day. In 2002, the National Academy of Sciences recommended 25 grams of fiber daily for women up to age 50 (slightly lower for women after age 50) and 38 grams a day for men. As registered dietitians, we see many patients who suffer from constipation, irritable bowel syndrome, elevated cholesterol levels, diabetes, and obesity. Many of these issues are related to low fiber intake.

What is Fiber?

Dietary fiber is the carbohydrate portion of plant foods that our bodies cannot digest or absorb. There are two kinds of dietary fiber: intact soluble and insoluble. Most foods contain some of both. Intact soluble fiber dissolves in water to form a gel-like, viscous substance. It can be found in oats, peas, beans, apples, citrus fruits, carrots, and barley. Insoluble fiber increases the movement of material through the digestive system. It is found in whole-wheat products, wheat bran, most vegetables, and nuts. Another type of insoluble fiber is resistant starch (RS). RS is a starch that "resists" digestion. Good sources include bananas, lentils, beans, and whole grains. Hi-maize resistant starch is made from special corn. It is added to certain products like Racconto pastas in an effort to increase fiber. It can also be purchased and added to cereals, smoothies, and baked products. For more information visit the websites: www.resistantstarch.com and www.hi-maize.com.

WHY IS FIBER GOOD FOR ME?

Fiber can help lower cholesterol levels, especially when combined with a low-fat diet. In fact, researchers at Harvard University found that men who consumed approximately 29 grams of fiber a day had a 40% reduction in heart attacks as compared to men with a low intake of fiber. Other studies have shown that a modest intake of fiber, about 10 grams a day, could increase the risk of a coronary event by 14% and coronary death by 27% when compared to a high fiber diet.

Fiber alters large bowel function by increasing the bulk of the stool and decreasing the amount of time it takes to move through the bowel. This process reduces the exposure of the bowel to carcinogens and protects against cancers of the colon and rectum. Fiber promotes regularity and may reduce the risk of diverticulitis—inflammation of small pouches in the lining of the colon.

Recommended adequate intake of Fiber: 38 grams for men and 25 grams for women per day.

Foods high in fiber will give you a sense of satiety —"full feeling" between meals-- and therefore aid in weight loss. In fact, the February 2011 Journal of

Nutrition reports a study of two groups of mice who had their calories restricted and then were allowed to eat as much as they wanted. One group of mice had fiber added to their diet. That group lost almost 4% of body fat. The other group regained their weight. So, adding more fiber to your diet may reduce the consumption of high calorie foods making it easier to lose weight.

What Can Fiber Do For You?

- Relieve constipation by forming the bulk of the stool and moving it faster through the GI tract
- Decrease your cholesterol, especially with a low-fat diet
- Alleviate irritable bowel syndrome
- Help those with diabetes control blood sugar levels
- Make you feel more full after eating, aiding in weight loss

WHOLE GRAINS

Whole grains are high in dietary fiber and vitamins, especially B vitamins, and are low in fat and cholesterol free. In order to get all the beneficial fiber and vitamins, all 3 parts of the grain must be consumed.

Refined grains have been processed to remove the bran and germ, leaving only the middle layer, which is devoid of most nutrients. Refined grains include white breads, rice, and flour. Processing removes approximately 25% of the grain's protein and as many as 17 different nutrients. Therefore, you should consume more whole grains as opposed to refined grains whenever possible. Try making at least half your grains whole grains. For cooking ideas see *Whole Grains for Busy People* by Lorna Sass.

Phytochemicals: Active chemical components present in a plant that account for its medicinal properties.

Whole grains contain a grain kernel that consists of 3 parts. These include:

1. **Outer bran: Rich in fiber**
2. **Middle endosperm: Makes up about 80% of the grain**
3. **Inner germ: Packed with nutrients**

Whole grain foods contain not only fiber but also hundreds of phytochemicals (such as phytoestrogens), antioxidants, phenols, vitamins, and minerals (such as Vitamin E and selenium). These may all play a role in disease prevention. Many of the compounds in grains, including antioxidants, have been shown to lower the risk factors for cardiovascular disease and some forms of cancer.

READING FOOD LABELS

Don't be fooled by the color of a product. Just because it has a caramel or brown color does not mean it is whole grain. For example, rye and pumpernickel bread seldom provide much fiber and definitely are not whole grain products, despite their dark color. The words "natural" and "organic" do not mean a food item is made from whole grains. Look for the words "whole wheat flour" on the ingredient list to be certain the product was made from the whole grain.

Look for food labels that have the following:

- <u>High fiber</u>—5 g or more per serving
- <u>Good source</u>—2.5 g to 4.9 grams per serving
- <u>More or added fiber</u>—At least 2.5 g per serving more than the reference food

---

Also, the number of grams of fiber on the label does not necessarily mean the food is whole grain. Whole grain products do have 2 grams of fiber or more in one serving; however, in order to determine if a product is truly whole grain, you must look on the label for the words "whole wheat" or "whole grain." Generally, a good source of fiber is any food that contains 2.5 or more grams of fiber per serving. Check the label and ingredient list for fiber information.

Some foods contain such foods such as inulin (aka chicory root extract), modified wheat starch, polydextrose, and maltodextrin. Inulin is added as "food" to prebiotics, to help boost intestinal flora. Modified wheat starch is an ingredient used in white, high fiber pasta, but there are no studies to date regarding the health benefit of this product. Although these are soluble fibers, they are not viscous or "gummy" and therefore have no effect in lowering cholesterol. These types of fiber are referred to in the world of food science as "isolated fiber" found in ice cream, yogurt, fat free half and half, white pastas, and some breakfast bars.

Naturally grown foods typically contain whole grains and most processed foods do not. However, there are some products that have added processed fiber, and they are a great healthy alternative. An example of this would be tapioca fiber that is processed and used as a fiber supplement in many foods. The fiber in these processed foods will still act as a laxative in preventing constipation, but remember that the antioxidants and phytonutrients that are only present in whole grains will be missing.

Some foods also contain the following functional fibers: cellulose, chitin, oligofrutose, fructoligosaccharides, lignin, pectins, psyllium, and inulin (aka chicory root). Besides being found in fruits and vegetables they are added to foods to increase fiber content. Inulin is often added to a large variety of foods such as candy bars, snack foods, and chocolate milk. Know that too much could cause gas and bloating.

FINDING HIGH FIBER FOODS

Adults should try to eat 25 – 35 grams of fiber each day. The key is to eat a variety of foods throughout the day, aiming for the recommended amount of each food group.

Breakfast

- Look for high-fiber cereals such as General Mill's Fiber One or Kellogg's All Bran containing as much as 13 grams of fiber in one serving.
- Add fruit on top of a high-fiber cereal and you could have half of your daily requirement in one meal!
- Try a 100% Whole Grain English Muffin.
- Try a homemade bran muffin along with a piece of fruit.

Lunch

- Look for Brownberry's or Pepperridge Farm's Whole Grain Bread with Double Fiber/Extra Fiber providing 6 grams of fiber per slice. That's an easy 12 grams for a sandwich.
- Add an apple for lunch and you'll have 14 grams for the meal.

Dinner

- Beans: Excellent source of fiber. They have soluble fiber, which can help lower cholesterol levels.
- Kidney beans, pinto beans, lentils, and black-eyed peas can be added to a salad, side dish, or bowl of soup.
- Canned beans are easy and fast, can be added to a meat or fish dish, or combined with rice.
- 1-cup serving of beans has as much as 10 to 13 grams of fiber.

Other Sources of Fiber

- Some new snack bars (be sure to read the label)
- Kraft Foods' line of 100% whole wheat crackers and cookies
- Flaxseed and bran can be added to yogurts or smoothies
- Mission or La Tortilla Factory whole grain tortilla wraps
- Fresh fruits and vegetables are easy portable snacks. Try throwing a few pieces of fruit, individual packages of raisins or cranberries, or some baby carrots in your briefcase or backpack.
- Benefiber® provides a natural source of soluble fiber that gently helps maintain regularity (information obtained from Mayo Clinic and the USDA National Nutrient Database). Each serving provides 3 grams of fiber and is easily mixed into beverages or soft foods. Try adding it to water, pudding, milk, cereal, yogurt, pasta sauce, or gelatin.
- Metamucil crackers also provides a natural source of fiber and helps maintain digestive health. Each serving contains 2 – 3 grams soluble fiber.

Here are a few tips to achieve the appropriate daily fiber goals in your diet:

- Start the day with a high fiber cereal, e.g., Fiber One or All Bran.
- Add fresh fruit to your cereal.
- Have a sandwich using whole grain bread, add lettuce, tomato, and a fresh fruit.
- Have ½ c of almonds or walnuts, or fresh fruit as an afternoon or morning snack.
- At dinner include a serving or two of vegetables and a baked potato or legumes.

If you total the amount of fiber contained in these high fiber foods, you will have reached your fiber target for the day (25-35 grams). With a little planning and smart shopping, meals and snacks can easily provide the right amount of fiber in your daily diet. Snack foods such as trail mix, nuts, fresh and dried fruits are portable and can be carried with you. Some of the new breakfast bars and sports bars also contain fiber. Remember, high fiber meals and snacks give you a "full" feeling and may help to reduce your overall calorie intake if you are trying to maintain or lose weight.

Be aware that increasing your fiber intake too quickly can cause intestinal gas, diarrhea, bloating, and intestinal discomfort, so increases should be done gradually. Begin by adding about 5 grams of fiber each week. Increase your water intake as you increase fiber because fiber can also cause constipation, or "binding" of fiber in the colon. Adding more fiber to your daily diet is a wise investment in your overall health.

> **Beware!** Begin fiber intake slowly; increase by 5 grams per day each week and increase water intake.

How much fiber is in the food I eat?

Check the fiber food list to see if you are getting 25-35 grams each day. Good sources of fiber have 2 grams or more fiber per serving. The following is a list of common foods and their fiber content.

Grains, Cereals, Pastas		
Food Item	**Serving size**	**Fiber Content**
All-Bran	½ cup	6.6g
Barley, pearled	1 cup	6g
Brown rice	1 cup	3.5g
Buckwheat, Soba Noodles	2 ounces	3g
Bulgur	1 cup	8g
Cheerios	1 cup	3g
Grape Nuts	½ cup	5g
Oatmeal, rolled	½ cup	5g
Quinoa	1 cup	4g
Raisin Bran	¾ cup	3g
Shredded Wheat	½ cup	4g
White rice	1 cup	0.6g
Whole wheat bread	1 slice	2g
Whole wheat spaghetti	1 cup	6.3g

Lentils, Beans, and Nuts		
Food Item	Serving size	Fiber content
Almonds	1 oz	3.3g
Baked beans	1 cup	16g
Black beans	1 cup	15g
Black-eyed peas	½ cup	3g
Cashews	1 oz	0.9g
Chickpeas	½ cup	5.3g
Great northern beans	½ cup	7g
Kidney beans	½ cup	6.5g
Lentils	1 cup	15.6g
Lima beans	½ cup	7g
Navy beans	½	9g
Peanuts	1 oz	2.4g
Peas, split (green)	1 cup	8g
Pinto beans	½ cup	7.3g
Pistachios	1 oz	2.9g
Soybeans (green)	½ cup	5g

Fruits		
Food Item	Serving size	Fiber content
Apple	1 medium	3.3g
Apricots, dried	8 halves	1g
Banana	1 medium	3.1g
Blackberries	½ cup	4g
Blueberries	1 cup	3.5g
Cantaloupe	1 wedge	0.6g
Figs	2 medium	3.7g
Grapes	1 cup	1.4g
Kiwifruit	1 fruit	2.3g
Orange	1 medium	3.1g
Papaya	1 cup	2.5g
Peach	1 medium	2.2g
Pear	1 medium	5.1g
Prunes	5 items	3g
Raspberries	½ cup	4g
Strawberries	1 cup	3.3g
Tomato	1 medium	1.5g
Watermelon	1 wedge	1.1g

Vegetables		
Food Item	**Serving size**	**Fiber content**
Artichoke	½ cup	4.5g
Asparagus, cooked	½ cup	1.8g
Baked potato w/skin	1 medium	4.4g
Baked sweet potato	1 medium	3.8g
Broccoli, raw	1 cup	2.4g
Brussels Sprouts, cooked	½ cup	2g
Cabbage, cooked	1 cup	3g
Carrots	1 medium	2g
Cauliflower, raw	½ cup	1.2g
Celery, raw	1 cup	1.6g
Collard greens	1 cup	1.5g
Corn	1 cup	3.2g
Cucumbers	10 slices	0.7g
Green beans, raw	1 cup	3.7g
Jicama, raw	½ cup	2.9g
Peas	1 cup	8.8g
Red bell pepper, raw	1 small	1.6g
Romaine Lettuce	1 cup	1g
Turnip greens	½ cup	2.5g
Winter squash, cooked	1 cup	5.7g

Information obtained from Mayo Clinic and the USDA National Nutrient Database and www.calorieking.com.

10 Reasons Dry Beans Promote Hearth Health

1. Dry beans contain no sodium.
2. Dry beans are a rich source of potassium.
3. Dry beans contain no cholesterol.
4. Dry beans are a fat-free food.
5. Dry beans are a rich source of dietary fiber, including cholesterol-binding soluble fiber.
6. Dry beans contain heart-healthy vegetable protein.
7. Dry beans are an excellent source of folic acid.
8. Dry bean consumption may help weight management.
9. People with diabetes who consume cooked, dry beans have a lower risk of heart disease.
10. Dry beans pair well with other heart health promoting foods like fish and virgin olive oil.

Maureen Murtaugh, PhD, RD
Dry Bean Quarterly
www.beaninstitute.com

Answers to Fiber Questions
1. True
2. True
3. True
4. False. High fiber foods can make you feel full and aid in weight loss efforts.
5. False. Women should eat 25 grams and men 38 grams daily.

CALCIUM

Check your understanding of Calcium by answering <u>True</u> or <u>False</u> to the following questions:

1. Men should not be concerned about calcium intake because they rarely have problems with bone density.
2. Consuming one glass of milk and one container of yogurt each day provides me with adequate calcium.
3. Calcium supplements should be taken between meals.
4. Osteoporosis is not a major issue in the United States.
5. Most of the calcium found in the body is stored in bones.
6. The most important dietary source of vitamin D is cheese.

Whether you're five, fifteen, or fifty, getting enough calcium in your diet is important. Adequate calcium intake can be a major concern for people who are always on the go because dairy products require refrigeration and are often unavailable. Yet new research has shown that individuals who consume adequate calcium are more likely to maintain a normal body weight. When you are running errands, picking up kids, or traveling for business, getting your daily requirement of calcium may take a little more effort than some of the other nutrients.

CALCIUM AND VITAMIN D

Before 18 years of age, our bone density has already been determined. The National Osteoporosis Foundation states that by our mid thirties bones slowly begin to lose their mass. After that time, our bodies need calcium to replenish calcium stores. While dairy products are the best sources of calcium, vitamin D plays a vital role in the absorption of calcium. Milk fortified with vitamin D is the most important source of calcium in our diet. Yogurt and cheese, which are good sources of calcium, are generally not fortified with vitamin D. Vitamin D can also be found in egg yolks, fortified margarines and butter, fortified cereals, fish liver oils, herring, and salmon.

Vitamin D can also be obtained from sunlight. Fifteen minutes in the direct sun, without sun block, can provide your daily vitamin D requirement. In colder climates, the amount of Vitamin D received from the sun is minimal so it is crucial to insure adequate dietary intake.

Factors that can reduce the amount of vitamin D obtained from sunlight

- Age
- Season
- Glass windows with UV protections
- Sunscreen use
- Latitude
- Clothing (especially covering the forearms)

There has been concern recently about the incidence of vitamin D deficiency. The National Health and Nutrition Examination Survey (NHANES) showed that few race, age, or gender groups meet the current dietary intake recommendations for vitamin D. It is estimated that 50% of the adult population is Vitamin D deficient. There is particular concern for individuals living in the colder climates. Reduced risk of these diseases can be associated with taking Vitamin D excess of the current recommendations.

Vitamin D Deficiency has been associated with

- Increased risk of heart disease
- Bone and muscle weakness
- High blood pressure
- Congestive heart failure
- Chronic blood vessel inflammation that is associated with hardening of the arteries
- Diabetes
- Certain cancers
- Multiple sclerosis

Vitamin D DRIs from the Food and Nutrition Board of the Institute of Medicine 2011	
Age group	**Dietary Reference Intake**
Infants 0-6 months	400 IU (10 mcg)
Infants 7-12 months	400 IU (10 mcg)
Children 1-3 years	600 IU (15 mcg)
Children 4-8 years	600 IU (15 mcg)
Children and Adults 9-70 years	600 IU (15 mcg)
Adults > 70 years	800 IU (20 mcg)
Pregnancy & Lactation	600 IU (15 mcg)

Calcium Recommendations from the Food and Nutrition Board of the Institute of Medicine 2011	
Age	**Dietary Reference Intake**
0-6 months	200 mg
7-12 months	260 mg
1-3 years	700 mg
4-8 years	1000 mg
9-18 years	1300 mg
Adults 19-50 years	1000 mg
Adults 51-70 years (M)	1000 mg
Adults 51-70 years (F)	1200 mg
Adults 71+ years	1200 mg
Postmenopausal or any amenorrheic women who is taking estrogen	1000 mg
Postmenopausal or any amenorrheic women who is not taking estrogen	1500 mg
Pregnant or breastfeeding women 14-18 years	1300 mg
Pregnant or breastfeeding women >19 years	1000 mg

The British Medical Journal reported that the use of calcium supplements needs to be reconsidered. This is due to a number of studies that showed the use of calcium supplements either with or without Vitamin D showed an increase in heart attacks. Dr. Mark J. Boland of the University of Auckland in New Zealand also questions the use of calcium supplements since they reduce fracture risk only marginally.

The American Academy of Pediatrics has recently recommended that all infants, children, and adolescents have a minimum daily vitamin D intake of 400 IU/day. These new guidelines are based on new clinical trials and for the prevention of rickets. The highest safe level for Vitamin D is 1,000 IU/day for infants 0-6 months, 1500 IU/day for infants 6-12 months, and 4000 IU/day for children through adults due to its toxic effects. Check the new Calcium and Vitamin Chart for more information.

Facts about Calcium

- The body gets the calcium it needs from the diet or takes what it needs from bones.
- Calcium is the most abundant mineral in the body; it is used to make bones and keep them strong.
- Ninety-nine percent of the calcium in the body is stored in the bones and teeth. The remainder of the body's calcium circulates in the blood and body tissues.
- This small amount of calcium allows muscle contraction, nerve conduction, blood clotting, iron utilization, activation of enzymes for metabolism, and regulation of nutrients in and out of cell walls.
- If there is not enough calcium in the blood and tissues, the body takes calcium from the bones to meet its needs. When this happens, the bones lose their strength and often break.
- During menopause and periods of amenorrhea, bone loss is accelerated due to the lack of the hormone estrogen, which affects the absorption of calcium. Adequate dietary intake of calcium can reduce the risk of bone loss.

IMPORTANT CONCERNS ABOUT CALCIUM ABSORPTION

Recent research suggests that drinking colas and other soft drinks may be bad for your bones. The American Journal of Clinical Nutrition reported the results of studies showing an association between soft drink intake and lower bone mineral density regardless of age, menopause, and calcium and vitamin D intake. When substituting soft drinks for milk, calcium and vitamin D intake can be compromised. Additionally, excessive caffeine consumption is linked to a higher risk of osteoporosis.

Studies have also shown that a diet high in sodium can rob the body of calcium. Other studies have shown that the lack of potassium and magnesium can be the culprits in reducing the body's supply of calcium. Dairy products are not only high in calcium, but also contain high levels of magnesium and potassium.

Calcium absorption can be affected by a number of factors	
Fiber	Adequate fiber intake is vital to keeping the digestive tract moving, reducing constipation, and decreasing the chance of diverticulosis (the formation of small pouches in the lining of the colon usually due to low fiber intake). However, large amounts of fiber, in particular bran, can decrease calcium absorption.
Protein	Adequate protein intake is crucial in calcium absorption, but excessive protein intake can increase urinary calcium excretion.
Meal Time	Some calcium supplements need to be taken with meals. This will ensure adequate calcium absorption by allowing stomach acids to dissolve and absorb the calcium. Be sure to read the supplement label for directions.
Caffeine	Drinking more than four cups of caffeinated coffee a day can increase calcium excretion. Also, soft drinks with caffeine can cause calcium loss.
Sodium	Excessive sodium consumption can increase urinary calcium excretion.
Green Leafy Vegetables	Oxalates and oxalic acid (found in green leafy vegetables) bind with calcium during digestion, making calcium insoluble. You can reduce these effects with adequate calcium intake.

The acid-base balance of the diet and its effect on bone and muscle health is an area that is being researched. Acid load contributed by the diet is not handled well by the elderly due to reduction in kidney function. The increase in acid concentration in the bloodstream causes muscle wasting because muscle and bone loss is the body's adaptation to excess acid. Grain products (bread, cereal, crackers, rice, and dessert items) increase acid levels. Fruits and vegetables are broken down to bicarbonate and add alkali to the body that neutralizes acid.

Another area of concern for risk of hip fracture is too much vitamin A retinol. Some research studies have found that very high doses of vitamin A can lead to massive bone loss and coma. To avoid this potential risk, vitamin A should be limited to 2000 to 3000 IU of retinol each day.

Osteoporosis is a condition that is characterized by a decrease of bone mass and bone density. The United States has one of the highest rates of osteoporosis in the world, with 15-20 million people affected and 80% of those people are women. Although osteoporosis is generally associated with post-menopausal women, over 2 million men also have been diagnosed with osteoporosis, and over 3 million men are at risk. It has been estimated that one out of eight men over the age of 50 will break a bone due to osteoporosis. The American Geriatric Society states that 20 to 24% of people who experience a hip fracture will die within the first year after the fracture. Adequate calcium intake is critically important to minimize these changes. (Check the exercise chapter for information on resistance and strength training exercises that help to enhance bone density.)

Six Other Bone-building Food Helpers

- Fish is an important addition to a bone-building diet due to its vitamin D content that helps absorb calcium. The best fish is salmon. A 3 ½ ounce serving will provide almost 90% of your daily vitamin D requirement.
- Seeds are an important source of magnesium that is found in healthy bones. Fifty percent of our body's magnesium is found in bones. All seeds provide magnesium, but pumpkin seeds are the highest source.
- Beans especially black, white, and kidney beans are high in magnesium and calcium. The US Dietary Guidelines for Americans recommends a weekly intake of 2 ½ cups of beans and other legumes. These would include peas and legumes.
- Nuts, especially walnuts, contain a rich source of alpha linolenic acid, an omega-3 fatty acid that helps in the reduction of bone breakdown and aids in bone formation.
- Leafy greens supply bone-building calcium, magnesium, and vitamin K. Vitamin K is crucial in the building of bones because they form bone proteins and cut calcium loss in the urine.
- Oysters contain our best source of zinc in the diet. Zinc helps in the formation of bone collagen that forms the protein framework of bones that allows them to be flexible.

DIETARY CALCIUM SOURCES

Good dietary sources of calcium include milk, yogurt, and cheese. Other non-dairy sources include tofu, sardines and salmon (with bones), almonds, broccoli, and collard greens. The charts that follow will show you some common sources of dietary calcium. Look on the label of most prepared products to find the % Daily Value calcium needs based upon a 2,000 calorie diet. When reading the label, check the label for the % Daily Value for calcium. If a food has 40% calcium, it contains 400 mg calcium (remove the % sign and add a zero).

Calcium in Foods
1000 mg Calcium
1 cup General Mills Raisin Bran Total cereal
¾ cup General Mill Whole grain Total cereal
1 1/3 cup Total Corn Flakes cereal
1 ¼ cup Harmony cereal * 600 mg
500 mg Calcium
I cup Lactaid Calcium-fortified milk
I packet Quaker Oatmeal Nutrition for Women

Calcium in Foods (Continued)
300-500 mg Calcium
1 cup skim or 2% milk
1 cup plain yogurt
1 cup orange juice fortified with calcium
1 cup cereal with 30% calcium
1 Sports bar with 30% calcium
1 cup Soy milk fortified with calcium (varies)
½ cup calcium enriched tofu
1 Starbucks Fat-free Tall Latte
1 ounce Kraft 2% grated cheddar cheese * 400 mg
Krusteaz Fat-Free Calcium Enriched Muffins
1 cup Ronzoni Smart Taste Pasta
200-300 mg Calcium
1 oz. most cheeses
1 slice calcium-enriched bread
1 cup 1% or 2% chocolate milk
1 cup macaroni and cheese
1 large slice cheese pizza
Fortified Cereal or Granola Bars (varies)
Instant Breakfast drink
Crystal-lite powdered drink mix enriched with Calcium
Minimum of 100 mg Calcium
½ cup broccoli
½ cup pudding
1 oz. Ricotta cheese
1 cup light ice cream or regular ice cream
½ cup tofu
3 oz. Canned salmon with bones
½ cup cooked collards
1 tbs. Blackstrap molasses
1 cup Cheerios (regular, Team, Frosted, Honey)
1 cup cereal with 10% calcium
2 Kellogg's Eggo Waffles
I can 7 up Plus soda

Diets rich in dairy foods have been shown to reduce the prevalence of metabolic syndrome in obese individuals. A prospective study of obese individuals in Caerphilly, UK, found men who regularly drank a pint of milk or more daily had reduced their odds of developing metabolic syndrome by 21%. However, the study did not find any significant trend for those with diabetes.

Calcium intake can be compromised by lactose intolerance. Nutrition Today (Sept. 2009) suggests that the prevalence of lactose intolerance may be lower than previously believed. If you feel lactose in milk causes you problems, try the National Dairy Council's tips to minimize problems with milk products:

DAIRY	
D	Drink milk with meals
A	Aged cheeses like cheddar and swiss are low in lactose
I	Introduce dairy slowly, gradually increase the amount consumed
R	Reduce lactose by enjoying lactose-free milk and milk products
Y	Yogurt with active cultures helps to digest lactose

Is refrigeration of dairy products causing you to avoid calcium? If so, try to meet your calcium needs with cheese on your sandwich, yogurt, or calcium-enriched food items. If you are unable to obtain low-fat yogurt and cheese when traveling or ordering lunch on the go, bring a calcium supplement with you to allow for your calcium needs while keeping your dietary intake lower in calories, fat, and cholesterol.

Calcium supplements come in a number of varieties:	
Calcium citrate	Calcium citrate is more readily absorbable. It can be taken at any time of the day and is not dependent on eating.
Calcium gluconate and Calcium lactate	Calcium gluconate and calcium lactate supplements contain less calcium per dose, making them more costly and less convenient.
Chelated calcium	Chelated supplements are not absorbed any better than other supplements; therefore, the additional cost is not justifiable.
Calcium phosphate	Calcium phosphate supplements should be avoided because the excess phosphorus could reduce calcium metabolism.
Oyster shell	Oyster shell supplements should be avoided because they may contain toxic contaminants such as lead.

Calcium supplements come in a number of varieties (continued):	
Cal-100 with D	Cal-100 with vitamin D provides 1000 mg of calcium and is found in a pre-measured, powdered form. Cal-100 is tasteless, non-gritty, and can be mixed with beverages or most solid foods. When mixed with orange juice, it produces a low acid, lightly carbonated beverage. This product is perfect for individuals who have problems swallowing large calcium tablets.
Calcium carbonate	Calcium carbonate is the most common calcium supplement. It can be found in chewable, capsule, tablet, and antacid forms. Viactiv is a popular chew that supplies 500mg calcium in each serving. Calcium carbonate needs to be taken twice a day at meals to meet the RDA for calcium. Be sure to take it with meals to ensure adequate calcium absorption by allowing stomach acid to be produced to dissolve and absorb the calcium.

The British Medical Journal reported that calcium supplement use needed to be reconsidered. Many studies have shown that calcium supplement use with or without Vitamin D showed an increase in heart attacks. Dr. Mark Boland of the University of Auckland in New Zealand also questions the use of calcium supplements because they reduce fracture risk marginally. The U.S. Preventative Services Task Force agreed with this position. They also found that supplementation in normal, healthy women also slightly increase the risk for kidney stones.

Answers to Calcium Questions

1. False. Men do need to worry about bone density. Over 2 million men have osteoporosis and over 3 million men are at risk in the United States.
2. False. Most people need more than a glass of milk and one container of yogurt each day to meet their calcium needs.
3. Calcium supplements are best taken with meals.
4. Osteoporosis is a major concern in the United States.
5. True
6. False. Milk is the best source of vitamin D in the diet.

ALCOHOL

> **"DRINK THE FIRST. SIP THE SECOND SLOWLY. SKIP THE THIRD." - KNUTE ROCKNE**

Test your Knowledge of Alcohol: Test your knowledge by responding <u>True</u> or <u>False</u> to the following questions.

1. Men should only consume 2 or fewer drinks a day and women should only consume 1 drink or fewer a day.
2. A serving of an alcoholic drink is 12 oz of beer, 5 oz of wine, or 1 ½ oz of spirits.
3. I do not have to worry about drinking alcohol when trying to lose weight because alcohol does not have many calories.
4. Alcohol can compromise a person's decision making by lowering the blood sugar level and dulling the senses.
5. Alcohol consumption during the cocktail hour can increase your consumption of food when the meal is served.
6. Alcohol has been implicated in some research studies for increasing cancer risk.

Whether you're celebrating an event, enjoying a before-dinner cocktail, or sipping a great Merlot, know the facts about alcohol. Alcoholic beverages are a common part of our social and business lives. Unfortunately alcohol supplies many empty calories and provides little nutrition. Excess alcohol can damage the body, especially the liver and brain.

The latest research recommends no more than two drinks per day for men and no more than one drink per day for women. One serving is equal to 12 oz of beer, 5 oz of wine, or 1 ½ oz of spirits. Women physiologically metabolize alcohol less efficiently than men. Men have 20 to 30 percent more water in their systems diluting the alcohol ingested.

Alcohol Servings:
1 Serving=1 ½ ounces spirits or 12 ounces beer or 5 ounces wine.

THE EFFECTS

The effects of alcohol are many and knowing them is important if you consume alcohol on a regular basis. Alcohol metabolism begins in the stomach and continues into the liver, where alcohol is metabolized. However, if alcohol consumption is too high and too fast for the liver to keep up, the alcohol will enter the blood system. This is when the adverse effects occur on many of our cells such as brain cells.

High in Calories
7 calories per gram of alcohol, 210 calories per ounce.

Alcohol is a diuretic and like any diuretic can cause dehydration if taken in large amounts. Alcohol can also irritate the stomach, making it a good idea to eat when drinking.

Alcohol ingestion causes a lowering of blood sugar levels, also known as hypoglycemia. It takes only two ounces of alcohol to produce hypoglycemia in a fasted person, which will also reduce inhibitions. The combination of low blood sugar and alcohol consumption can make us hungrier as well. When consuming cocktails, munching on appetizers and enjoying the company of others, it is common to lose track of what we eat and drink causing us to overdo it. Alcohol is relatively high in calories; there are 7 calories per gram of alcohol. If those extra calories are not burned up in the form of exercise, they are stored as fat. Although the cocktail hour is a common American custom, it is far better to eat before drinking to avoid the effects of alcohol consumption. These effects include: increased hunger, increased consumption of food, and increased storage of fat.

Also know that how quickly you down that drink affects the rate at which alcohol is absorbed into your bloodstream, and how intoxicated you will feel. A martini sipped over an hour will have the same effect as a glass of wine drunk in a half hour. Research also showed that individuals who had a bubbly or carbonated drink may feel the effects of alcohol sooner rather than later.

THE ADVANTAGES

The good news is that research has shown that moderate intake of beer, wine, or spirits can aid in protecting the heart. This happens because alcohol can reduce the "stickiness" of blood that can contribute to blood clots. Another study showed that individuals who had one to six drinks a week had higher levels of HDL cholesterol, the "good" cholesterol.

Red wine has a phytochemical called resveratrol. Studies have shown that resveratrol prevents clotting and plaque formation in the arteries. Red wine contains more resveratrol than white wine. The amount of resveratrol in wine depends upon the amount of time the skin of the grape is left on while making the wine. In the case of white wine, the skin is removed before the fermentation so it has a lower concentration. Resveratrol can also be found in grape juice (the purple grape juice), red grapes, cocoa, dark chocolate, peanuts, blueberries, mulberries, and is also sold as a supplement.

THE DISADVANTAGES

- A 50% increase in the risk of hypertension was reported in a study from 2004, State University of New York at Buffalo in those individuals who drank alcohol without food.
- Drinking one alcoholic beverage a day increased a woman's breast cancer risk by 10 to 30%, according to American Cancer society senior epidemiologist Heather Spencer Feigelson, PhD.
- Since alcohol dilates blood vessels over time, too much drinking can stretch the capillaries, giving your face a permanent red hue, says David Colbert, a New York City dermatologist.

HANGOVER HELP

For some, it might take just a glass or two of red wine; for others, they may consume too many drinks to remember. Regardless of the amount of alcohol, a hangover is a hangover, leaving one feeling miserable the day after. Mayo Clinic recommends sipping a glass of water between drinks to avoid dehydration. Another tip is to drink a glass of water before bed and in the morning upon awakening. If you are dehydrated, it's a good idea to eat foods high in salt and potassium. Try some salty soup and fruit or fruit juices. Orange and grapefruit juice and bananas are good sources of potassium. If stomach upset is present, avoid spicy foods.

THE CULPRIT

Congeners are chemicals found in dark colored drinks. They add color and flavor and are more apt to cause a hangover. Light colored beverages, such as vodka, gin, and light beers are less likely to cause hangover effects than dark colored drinks.

Here's a list of drinks with high levels of congeners

- Bourbon
- Brandy
- Dark-colored beers and beer with a high alcohol content

- Red wine
- Scotch
- Tequila

Simple Tips for Alcohol Use

- Limit alcohol consumption to two alcoholic beverages per day, once to twice each week.
- Consume a snack such as fruit or crackers before you drink to prevent low blood sugar that can cause hunger and over-eating.
- Limit drinks that contain large quantities of sugar such as liqueurs, sweet wines, fruit juice, soda pop, tonic water, or drink mixes.
- Sugar-free soda pop or drink mixes and soda water are healthier choices and reduce calories and sugar significantly.

- Light beer is preferable to regular beer and ale because of the lower carbohydrate content (3-6 grams versus 15 grams per can).
- Remember to count the calories from alcohol as part of your daily intake.
- Cut down your use of alcohol by drinking a diet drink or water between each alcoholic beverage consumed.
- Switch to a Shirley Temple or "mocktail" after a drink or two; a spritzer with a small amount of juice is a good substitute.
- Drink your beverages slowly.

Alcohol Content		
Beverage (amount)	Calories	Carbohydrate (grams)
Non-alcoholic beer 12 oz	70	17.5
Light beer 12 oz	100	4.8
Regular beer 12 oz	146	13.2
Gin 94-proof 1.5 oz	124	0
Rum 94-proof 1.5 oz	124	0
Vodka 94-proof 1.5 oz	124	0
Whiskey 94-proof 1.5 oz	124	0
Whiskey Sour 4 oz	170	0
Dessert Wine 3.5 oz	150	12
Red Wine 3.5 oz	72	3
White Wine 3.5 oz	70	2
Rose Wine 3.5 oz	70	1
Gin & Tonic*	188	16
Rum & Coke *	201	20
7&7 *	196	18
Vodka cranberry *	251	31
Red bull & vodka *	311	20.2
Margarita *	105	10.8
Vodka Tonic *	188	16
Vodka & orange juice*	174	18.4
Long Island Iced Tea*	196	0
Amaretto Stone Sour*	283	29
Martini*	156	0.2
Classic	139	0.4
Apple	235	11.6
Chocolate	438	24
Jack Daniels & Coke*	201	20
Manhattan*	128	1.8

*Drinks include 1.5 oz of alcohol

Answers to Alcohol Questions

1. True.
2. True.
3. False.   Alcohol provides 7 calories per gram of ethanol.   This is more energy than what carbohydrates and protein provide.
4. True.
5. True.
6. True.

CAFFEINE

Check your understanding of Caffeine by answering <u>True</u> or <u>False</u> to the following questions:

1. Coffee is the highest caffeine-containing food product.

2. Caffeine is addictive.

3. I can use caffeine to lose weight because it decreases my appetite.

4. There are no adverse effects to consuming caffeine products.

5. The recommended intake of caffeine is less than 300 mg per day.

Whether it's a morning cup of coffee or an afternoon pick me up, most of us can't imagine starting our day without a cup of coffee. Coffee is the highest caffeine-containing food. Other items include: tea, cola, energy drinks, chocolate, and some prescription and non-prescription drugs.

People continue to consume a considerable amount of caffeine throughout the day. Coffee is the highest caffeine-containing food product, and its availability during the day easily contributes to its high consumption.

FACTS ABOUT CAFFEINE

Caffeine is found naturally in various plants, acting as a mild stimulant. Although caffeine is not addictive, it can be habit forming. When stopped abruptly, individuals experience headaches, irritability, fatigue, and/or drowsiness.

Within five minutes of ingestion, caffeine begins to stimulate the central nervous system which responds by releasing stress hormones. This may cause a short increase in alertness, usually followed by agitation. As the levels of stress hormones diminish, individuals feel hungry and more tired. This often results in the consumption of another cup of coffee or cola containing caffeine. Since hunger is then stimulated, a high-sugar snack may also accompany the caffeine-containing beverage. Although this combination of items may give temporary energy, it can also cause exhaustion and an inability to focus later in the day.

HEALTH CONCERNS

Experts advise us to limit caffeine intake to less than 300 mg daily, which is equivalent to approximately 16 ounces of coffee. Check out your caffeine intake by reviewing the caffeine content chart at the end of this chapter. When lowering caffeine, start by monitoring the effects of your current intake. Then, slowly start to cut your intake down. Cutting out caffeine too abruptly can cause side effects, similar to those probably experienced when you "missed" your morning coffee or cola.

Be aware of the effects caffeine can have on your performance at home and at work. When meetings and meals out are accompanied with cola or coffee, make sure the extra caffeine is not compromising your work performance or general sense of well-being. A high caffeine intake can cause irritability, fatigue, agitation, or anxiety. If any of these symptoms are a concern, consider cutting down on your caffeine intake. Luckily, there are plenty of ways to reduce your caffeine intake. Suggestions are covered at the end of this chapter.

Individuals with a family history of heart disease, hypertension, and osteoporosis are wise to reduce or eliminate their caffeine consumption. Persons with a history of ulcers should omit caffeine entirely from their diet, because it causes an increase in stomach acid, which can aggravate an ulcer.

Caffeine is a diuretic that increases the elimination of fluids from the body, which can result in dehydration and calcium loss. When adequate hydration is important, such as athletic events or when spending the day outdoors, caffeine consumption should be carefully monitored. Pregnancy or sports participation requires a special need for adequate fluid intake. When caffeine is consumed, more non-caffeinated fluids may be required to make up for the fluid lost. Many pregnant women or athletes find that it is wiser to eliminate caffeine completely.

Caffeine sensitivity varies from person to person. For example, individuals with shorter stature may feel caffeine's effects more strongly than heavier, taller individuals.

CAFFEINE'S EFFECTS

The effects of caffeine have been associated with elevated blood sugar levels, increased lipid levels, blood pressure, heart rate, urination, irritability, constriction of blood vessels, increased anxiety, insomnia, and decreased absorption of iron, zinc, calcium, potassium, magnesium, and sodium.

Research studies have attempted to link the use of caffeine to an increased risk for heart disease, hypertension, cancer, high cholesterol, osteoporosis, and fibrocystic breast disease. However, research is on-going and no firm evidence has yet established that caffeine intake is associated with these conditions. Moderate caffeine intake (300 mg of caffeine per day) has not been shown to increase either the chances of infertility or a pregnancy outcome.

Don't give up on that cup of coffee yet. There are some positive benefits from coffee consumption! Recent Harvard research has shown that consuming 1-3 cups of coffee daily can reduce Type II diabetes. When more than 6 cups of coffee were consumed daily, men's diabetes risk was reduced by 54% and women's risk by 30% compared to non-coffee drinkers.

Tomas De Paul, a Ph.D. research scientist at Vanderbilt University Institute, has done a number of coffee studies. He has found that regular coffee drinkers are 80% less likely to develop Parkinson's disease. Other research has shown that consuming at least 2 cups of coffee daily can reduce colon cancer risk by 25%, liver cirrhosis by 80%, and gallstones by 50%.

Evidence has also shown that coffee may reduce asthma symptoms, stop headaches, elevate mood, and prevent cavities. The compound that gives coffee its aroma and bitter taste has been found to be responsible for its antibacterial and adhesive properties that prevent dental cavities from forming.

When reducing caffeine intake, start with the following suggestions

- Limit caffeine intake to no more than 200-300 mg each day, about two cups of coffee (8 ounces each).

- Drink half decaffeinated coffee or colas and half regular coffee or colas.

- Substitute with decaffeinated beverages and herbal teas.

- Eat meals at regular times with no more than four hours between each meal.

- Quit smoking, since smoking and drinking coffee often go together.

- Get adequate sleep.

- Establish a regular exercise schedule. Run, walk, bike, swim, yoga, meditate.

- Choose healthier foods. Fatty foods and alcohol can make you drag, causing you to respond with a caffeinated beverage.

A new trend is the use of energy drinks by young people to boost their energy. In November 2011, the Federal Substance Abuse and Mental Health Services Department reported that since 2005, emergency room visits for energy drink use has risen ten-fold in the U.S. Forty-four percent of young adults are also combining the use of energy drinks with alcohol and drugs. Kids are coming into the emergency room with heart palpitations, light headedness, dizziness, headaches, and feeling faint. Young adults may be placing themselves at risk due to the fact that energy drinks may contain three times the caffeine as colas. Mixing energy drinks with booze is particularly dangerous. This is because the caffeine keeps them awake, allowing them to drink much more. Dr. Tom Scaletta, the director of Edward's Hospital emergency room in Naperville, IL, finds these young adults unarousable due to the amount of alcohol they've drunk.

Many people are unaware of the amount of caffeine they consume daily. It is important to recognize the adverse effects of caffeine and adjust your intake accordingly. Caffeine should be avoided completely if health concerns are an issue and always consult with your physician and dietitian to make a plan specific to your needs. As with all foods, moderation is the key.

Caffeine Content of Foods and Drugs		
OTC Drugs	**Serving Size**	**Caffeine (mg)**
NoDoz, maximum strength; Vivarin	1 tablet	200
Excedrin	2 tablets	130
NoDoz, regular strength	1 tablet	100
Anacin	2 tablets	64
Coffee	**Serving Size**	**Caffeine (mg)**
Coffee, brewed	8 ounces	135
Coffee, expresso	2 ounces	120
General Foods International Coffee, Orange Cappuccino	8 ounces	102
Coffee, instant	8 ounces	95
Coffee, instant decaffeinated	8 ounces	2
General Foods International Coffee, Cafe Vienna	8 ounces	90
Maxwell House Cappuccino, Mocha	8 ounces	60-65
General Foods International Coffee, Swiss Mocha	8 ounces	55
Maxwell House Cappuccino, French Vanilla or Irish Cream	8 ounces	45-50
Maxwell House Cappuccino, Amaretto	8 ounces	25-30
General Foods International Coffee, Viennese Chocolate Cafe	8 ounces	26
Maxwell House Cappuccino, decaffeinated	8 ounces	6-Mar
Coffee, decaffeinated	8 ounces	5
Tea	**Serving Size**	**Caffeine (mg)**
Celestial Seasonings Iced Lemon Ginseng Tea	16-ounce bottle	100
Bigelow Raspberry Royale Tea	8 ounces	83
Tea, leaf or bag	8 ounces	50
Iced Tea	12 ounces	70
Mint Tea	8 ounces	50
Oolong Tea	8 ounces	40
Orange and Spice	8 ounces	45
Snapple Iced Tea, all varieties	16-ounce bottle	42

Tea	Serving Size	Caffeine (mg)
Lipton Natural Brew Iced Tea Mix, unsweetened	8 ounces	25-45
Lipton Tea	8 ounces	35-40
Lipton Iced Tea, assorted varieties	16-ounce bottle	18-40
Lipton Natural Brew Iced Tea Mix, sweetened	8 ounces	15-35
Nestea Pure Sweetened Iced Tea	16-ounce bottle	34
Tea, green	8 ounces	30
Arizona Iced Tea, assorted varieties	16-ounce bottle	15-30
Lipton Soothing Moments Blackberry	Tea 8 ounces	25
Nestea Pure Lemon Sweetened Iced Tea	16-ounce bottle	22
Tea, instant	8 ounces	15
Lipton Natural Brew Iced Tea Mix, diet	8 ounces	10-15
Lipton Natural Brew Iced Tea Mix, decaffeinated	8 ounces	< 5
Celestial Seasonings Herbal Tea, all varieties	8 ounces	0
Celestial Seasonings Herbal Iced Tea, bottled	16-ounce bottle	0
Lipton Soothing Moments Peppermint Tea	8 ounces	0
Soft Drinks	**Serving Size**	**Caffeine (mg)**
Josta	12 ounces	58
Mountain Dew	12 ounces	55.5
Surge	12 ounces	52.5
Diet Coke	12 ounces	46.5
Coca-Cola classic	12 ounces	34.5
Dr. Pepper, regular or diet	12 ounces	42
Squirt Ruby Red	12 ounces	90
Mello Yellow	12 ounces	53
Sunkist Orange Soda	12 ounces	42
Pepsi-Cola	12 ounces	37.5
Barqs Root Beer	12 ounces	22.5
7-UP or Diet 7-UP	12 ounces	0
Barqs Diet Root Beer	12 ounces	0

Soft Drinks Continued	Serving Size	Caffeine (mg)
Caffeine-free Coca-Cola or Diet Coke	12 ounces	0
Caffeine-free Pepsi or Diet Pepsi	12 ounces	0
Minute Maid Orange Soda	12 ounces	0
Mug Root Beer	12 ounces	0
Sprite or Diet Sprite	12 ounces	0
Energy Drinks	**Serving Size**	**Caffeine (mg)**
Red Bull	8.3 ounces	80
Amp	16 ounces	143
Full Throttle Energy	16 ounces	144
Rockstar	16 ounces	160
Caffeinated Water	**Serving Size**	**Caffeine (mg)**
Java Water	1/2 liter (16.9 ounces)	125
Krank 20	1/2 liter (16.9 ounces)	100
Aqua Blast	1/2 liter (16.9 ounces)	90
Water Joe	1/2 liter (16.9 ounces)	60-70
Aqua Java	1/2 liter (16.9 ounces)	50-60
Juice	**Serving Size**	**Caffeine (mg)**
Juiced	10 ounces	60
Java Juice	12 ounces	90
Frozen Desserts	**Serving Size**	**Caffeine (mg)**
Ben & Jerry's No Fat Coffee Fudge Frozen Yogurt	1 cup	85
Starbucks Coffee Ice Cream, assorted flavors	1 cup	40-60

Frozen Desserts Continued	Serving Size	Caffeine (mg)
Häagen-Dazs Coffee Ice Cream	1 cup	58
Häagen-Dazs Coffee Frozen Yogurt, fat-free	1 cup	40
Häagen-Dazs Coffee Fudge Ice Cream, low-fat	1 cup	30
Starbucks Frappuccino Bar	1 bar (2.5 ounces)	15
Healthy Choice Cappuccino Chocolate Chunk or Cappuccino Mocha Fudge Ice Cream	1 cup	8
Yogurt, one container	**Serving Size**	**Caffeine (mg)**
Dannon Coffee Yogurt	8 ounces	45
Yoplait Cafe Au Lait Yogurt	6 ounces	5
Dannon Light Cappuccino Yogurt	8 ounces	< 1
Stonyfield Farm Cappuccino Yogurt	8 ounces	0
Chocolates or Candies	**Serving Size**	**Caffeine (mg)**
Hershey's Special Dark Chocolate Bar	1 bar (1.5 ounces)	31
Perugina Milk Chocolate Bar with Cappuccino Filling	1/3 bar (1.2 ounces)	24
Hershey Bar (milk chocolate)	1 bar (1.5 ounces)	10
Coffee Nips (hard candy)	2 pieces	6
Cocoa or Hot Chocolate	8 ounces	5
Chocolate Chips	1 cup	104

Sources for table:

- Serving sizes are based on commonly eaten portions, pharmaceutical instructions, or the amount of the leading-selling container size. For example, beverages sold in 16-ounce or half-liter bottles were counted as one serving.

- National Coffee Association, National Soft Drink Association, Tea Council of the USA, and information provided by food, beverage, and pharmaceutical companies and J.J.

- Barone, H.R. Roberts (1996) "Caffeine Consumption." *Food Chemistry and Toxicology*, vol. 34, pp. 119-129.

- Bowes &Church's Food Values of Portions Commonly Used. 17th Edition, J.B. Lippincott Company, 1994, pg. 381-383.

Answers to Caffeine Questions:

1. True.

2. False. Caffeine is not addictive but it is habit forming.

3. False. Caffeine will stimulate hunger so using caffeine as a weight loss method will most likely not lead to the results you want.

4. False. The adverse effects of caffeine are irritability, tiredness, anxiety, hunger, and inability to focus.

5. True.

PREBIOTICS AND PROBIOTICS

Both prebiotics and probiotics have been touted as having many health benefits. Prebiotics, also known as fermentable fibers, are non-digestible and naturally occurring food ingredients that stimulate the growth or activity of probiotics activity. As prebiotics are processed through the digestive tract and fermented in the colon, they encourage the growth of "healthy" gut bacteria. The 2009 Diabetes Care and Education Dietetic Practice Group of The Academy of Nutrition and Dietetics states that there are many benefits to using prebiotics as part of your daily diet.

There is no recommended daily value for prebiotics. Prebiotics can be found in a variety of foods and are also available in supplements that include powder, capsules, tablets, and drops. The two most common prebiotics are inulin and oligofructose. Inulin is found in a variety of foods including: artichokes, asparagus, onions, garlic, bananas, wheat, rye, and chicory root. Oligofructose is found in fruits. Two other prebiotics are resistant starch and galacto-oligosaccharide. These starches are found naturally in raw potatoes, cooked and cooled starchy foods, and unripe bananas. They are also found in some varieties of packaged pasta, dairy and bakery items, cereals and cereal bars, and some table spreads.   Know that companies don't have to tell you how much is in a product.

You can find more information by visiting these websites: International Food Information Council and International Scientific Association for Probiotics and Prebiotics:
 www.isapp.net and the International Food Information Council: www.ific.org

- Maintains a healthy digestive system.

- Allows beneficial bacteria to grow in place of harmful bacteria in the intestine.

- Strengthens the body's natural defenses.

- Improves bowel function.

- Increases mineral absorption of calcium, iron, and magnesium.

- May have a cholesterol lowering affect.

PROBIOTICS

Probiotics, also known as bifidobacteria and lactobacilli, are live bacteria that enhance your natural immune system and promote intestinal health and regularity. They are eaten as part of fermented foods that have live and active cultures. The most commonly known one is lactobacillus acidophilus found in yogurt. When you read labels make sure it says "live and active" culture, e.g., lactobacillus. Some fermented foods that contain these bacteria are yogurt, soy drinks, miso, sauerkraut, fermented and unfermented milk.

Research is limited on the benefits but preliminary findings have shown positive benefits. Side effects include gas and bloating.

Foods Containing Prebiotics

• artichokes	• flax
• bananas	• greens: chard and kale
• barley	• honey
• berries	• legumes
• chicory	• onions
• dairy products	• wheat and whole grain

FOOD ALLERGIES

Food allergies are often confusing and misunderstood. Too often we hear about individuals restricting certain foods or food groups based on their assumption that they are allergic to that food or nutrient. A true food allergy triggers the body to produce an immunologic response to a particular food. Even trace amounts of a food allergen can cause a reaction.

The symptoms described by individuals complaining of a food allergy are often not scientifically supported. Unfortunately foods are unnecessarily eliminated from the diet and in extreme cases nutrition is compromised.

In severe cases the following symptoms may occur

- Constriction of airways
- Swollen throat or sensation of a lump in your throat
- Difficulty breathing
- Shock, severe drop in blood pressure
- Dizziness, lightheadedness or a sudden loss of consciousness
- If not immediately treated can result in coma or death.

The 2009 Journal of The Academy of Nutrition and Dietetics states that about 4 percent to 8 percent of children under the age of 18 and 2 percent of adults have food allergies. The Guidelines for the Diagnosis and Management of Food Allergies in the U.S. lists the most common food allergies as peanut, tree nuts, wheat, crustacean shellfish, and soy.

The National Institute of Allergy and Infectious Disease (NIAID) of the National Institutes of Health organized a group of experts to set up guidelines. The Recommendations for diagnosing a food allergy are the following:

- In-depth medial history and physical
- Skin Prick Test – should be used to diagnosis a skin allergy
- Food Elimination Diets – may be used for Oral Food Challenges

This report also states that the double-blinded placebo- controlled food challenge is considered the gold standard. One blood test or skin test is not sufficient to make a diagnosis of a true food allergy.

There are some tests used that are not reliable and not recommended for diagnosing food allergies.

- Basal histamine release/activation
- Lymphocyte stimulation
- Facial thermography
- Gastric juice analysis
- Endoscopic allergen provocation
- Hair analysis applied kinesiology
- Provocation neutralization
- Allergen-specific IgG4
- Cytotoxicity assays
- Electrodermal test (Vega)
- Mediator release assay (Leap diet)

If you suspect a food allergy contact your physician before making changes in your diet. A board-certified allergist can confirm a food allergy and a registered dietitian can help with the eating challenges that present.

Though eating out can be a challenge for individuals with food allergies, many restaurants train staff to accommodate individuals with food allergies. The Food Allergy Buddy Dining Card was developed to inform restaurant staff and chefs of any specific food allergy. It is available for free at www.foodallergybuddy.com. The Food Allergy and Anaphylaxis Network (FAAN) and the National Restaurant Association have developed a training program for restaurants to increase awareness of food allergies.

The following tips can make eating out safer and worry free:

- Phone ahead and notify the chef and wait staff of your allergy.

- Check out the menu ahead of time if the restaurant has a website.

- Ask the chef for menu ideas that will eliminate the know allergen.

- When you arrive at the restaurant remind the wait staff of your allergy.

- Be aware of hidden ingredients in sauces, dressings, stuffing, breading, and baked goods. Know the alternative names for your specific allergy.

- Use the Food Allergy Buddy Dining Card program to inform restaurant staff of a food allergy.

- Bring "Allernotes", which are preprinted sticky notes listing your food allergy, that the server can attach to your order.

- Be aware of cross contact from cooking oils, splatter, and steam from cooking foods or utensils that come into contact with food allergens.

- If traveling to a foreign country you can create for $10 a food allergy card in your native language that automatically translates into any language you choose.

- Carry your food allergy medications with you at all times. Let those that you are with know about your food allergy.

- Make sure that you check to see how their meat is raised. Meats marked as natural or vegetarian fed may have been fed corn or soy.

For our patients with severe food allergies, we have found the following suggestions to be helpful:

- Check botanical food family lists. For individuals with a food or plant allergy, they may be sensitive to foods or plants in the same botanical group. An example would be green peas from the legume list. Those with a green pea allergy might also be allergic to other items in the legume list.

- Corn is present in practically everything. Be careful with items with glucose, dextrose, food starch etc. that contain hidden corn.

- Do not buy foods that are not labeled and read the entire label from front to back.

- Do not buy foods from bins due to the possibility of cross-contamination.

- Medications, toothpaste, cosmetics, and toiletries can contain foods that cause allergies.

- Avoid most deli meats since they often have one machine that slices the meats leading to cross-contamination.

- Individuals allergic to corn need to watch for citric acid. It is made from mold fed sugar solutions that are often derived from corn.

Helpful resources include: The Webstaurant Store website, Eating with Food Allergies, WebMD, and the National Restaurant Association.

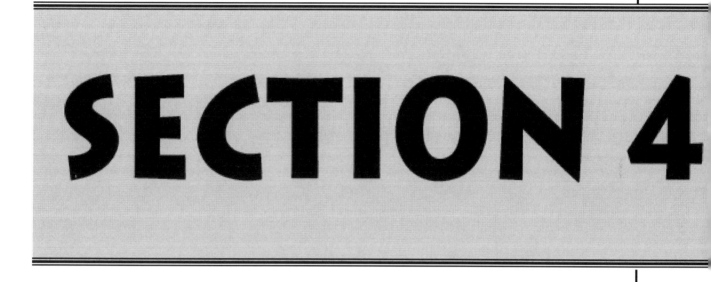

SECTION 4

QUICK & EASY FOOD PLANNING & PREPARATION

Meal Planning

1. Make out your week's menus using the Weekly Menu Planning Guide.
2. Plan menus weekly to save time when shopping. Having enough food on hand allows only occasional trips to the store for perishables.
3. When planning menus, check newspaper ads for weekly sale items that can be used for meals to allow money saving.
4. Consider the use of store shopping programs that will deliver your food to your home, like Pea Pod grocery shopping service. This will save you time and reduce impulse buying.
5. Pick the correct number of servings from the five major food groups when planning your daily menus. Use www.ChooseMyPlate.gov, www.mealsmatter.org, and www.foodonthetable.com to guide your food selection.
6. Using a menu helps you to plan on using leftovers more effectively. For example, if you serve turkey or ham on Saturday, you can plan on the use of soups, sandwiches, or casseroles for meals during the week. Some of these items could be made on Sundays or put together quickly during the week. This is particularly useful for late nights at work when fatigue leads to impulse eating.
7. Select an entrée for each lunch and dinner. Use foods on hand to complement each meal.
8. Review the Snack Chapter for healthy snacks, adding these to your shopping list on page 158.

Weekly Menu Planning Guide

	Sunday	Monday	Tuesday	Wednesday	Thursday	Friday	Saturday
Breakfast							
Fruit or juice							
Cereal or Starch							
Protein							
Beverage and/or milk							

	Sunday	Monday	Tuesday	Wednesday	Thursday	Friday	Saturday
Lunch							
Entrée							
Vegetable							
Starch							
Fruit							
Beverage and/or milk							

	Sunday	Monday	Tuesday	Wednesday	Thursday	Friday	Saturday
Dinner							
Entrée							
Vegetable							
Starch							
Fruit							
Beverage and/or milk							
Salad							
Dessert							

SHOPPING

"DON'T EAT ANYTHING YOUR GREAT-GREAT GRANDMOTHER WOULDN'T RECOGNIZE AS FOOD. THERE ARE A GREAT MANY FOOD-LIKE ITEMS IN THE SUPERMARKET YOUR ANCESTORS WOULDN'T RECOGNIZE AS FOODS. STAY AWAY FROM THESE". MICHAEL POLLAN.

Grocery shopping trends have changed in the last 25 years. Surveys show that between 30-60% of men are doing the primary shopping, up from 14% in 1985. Whether this is due to more men being laid off from work or more couples sharing household duties, men's contribution to shopping has had a major impact. Some characteristics of the male shopper include:

- Tend to walk through all of the aisles exploring different food options.
- Spend more time shopping and are less hurried.
- Apt to impulse buy.
- Enjoy customizing and adding a personal touch.
- Appear to be more experimental and adventurous in their food purchasing.
- Shop around the store for the best price more than women.
- Ask for help less often and generally make a second sweep through the store.

Regardless of your shopping style, use the Weekly Menu Planning Guide first to save time and make the best food decisions.

To make the best use of your time, plan your week of meals using the Weekly Menu Planning Guide first. Then, check the foods you have on hand and use your shopping list to organize the foods you need. Take into consideration meal planning if you will be eating at home or on the road. Fill in the out of town meals with ideas of what you will order when you are away. This will help you stick to your nutrition plan, because planning ahead will reduce impulse ordering. When you've completed your meal plans for four separate weeks you'll notice quite a variety of foods. If you don't, review the menus for the month and change some of the meals to provide different items. Planning a month of meal plans will allow variety and give you the ability to use them over and over again. At times, you may want to add new items that can be substituted for your favorites to prevent boredom with your meals.

1. Keep a running shopping list each week and add items to your list as your supplies run low.
2. Use a shopping list that is arranged by categories. This will reduce your shopping time if you use the list to correspond to the traffic pattern of your favorite store.
3. Use seasonal fresh fruits and vegetables to keep your costs down.
4. Eat before shopping to reduce impulse buying caused by hunger.
5. Leave the kids home, if possible, to avoid food fights in the store and excessive demands that cost you more money.
6. If you can't leave the kids at home, beware of pressures to buy candy, cookies, or other treats in order to appease a complaining child. Bring lower calorie choices to the store with you that they can snack on. These would include: fresh fruit, graham crackers, pretzels, or popcorn.
7. Cross off items as you select them. Sticking to your lists will reduce impulse buying. Check labels to insure the purchase of the best buy. Ingredients must be listed in the order that they predominate. Example: A label listing water, gravy, potatoes, carrots, and beef contains the most water and the least amount of beef.
8. Pass items at the check-out and at waist level since they are designed for impulse buying.
9. Purchase packages based upon how quickly you're able to use them. Usually a larger package is more economical, unless it can't be used or stored before it spoils.
10. If you have problems limiting portion sizes, buy individual serving snack packs. When you are done with the package it is a reminder that you have eaten your allotted amount.
11. Shop for packaged goods and staples first. Shop for perishable foods and frozen food last. As you unpack your order put away perishables first. Always move older supplies forward and put new supplies in the back of your storage area.
12. Shop on days when foods are freshest and most plentiful, usually toward the end of the week.

The Shopping List

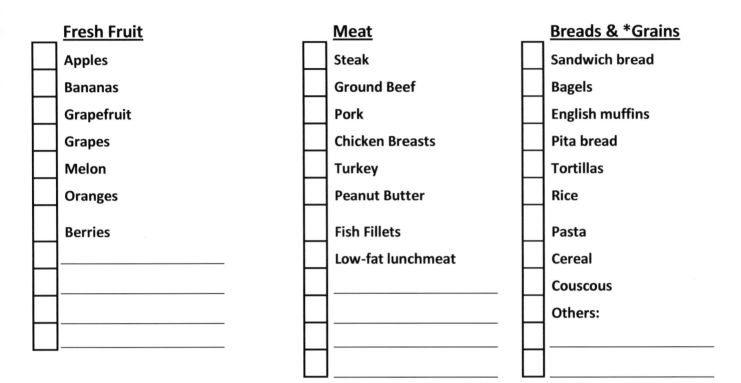

Fresh Fruit

- [ ] Apples
- [ ] Bananas
- [ ] Grapefruit
- [ ] Grapes
- [ ] Melon
- [ ] Oranges
- [ ] Berries
- [ ] _____
- [ ] _____
- [ ] _____
- [ ] _____

Meat

- [ ] Steak
- [ ] Ground Beef
- [ ] Pork
- [ ] Chicken Breasts
- [ ] Turkey
- [ ] Peanut Butter
- [ ] Fish Fillets
- [ ] Low-fat lunchmeat
- [ ] _____
- [ ] _____
- [ ] _____

Breads & *Grains

- [ ] Sandwich bread
- [ ] Bagels
- [ ] English muffins
- [ ] Pita bread
- [ ] Tortillas
- [ ] Rice
- [ ] Pasta
- [ ] Cereal
- [ ] Couscous
- [ ] Others:
- [ ] _____

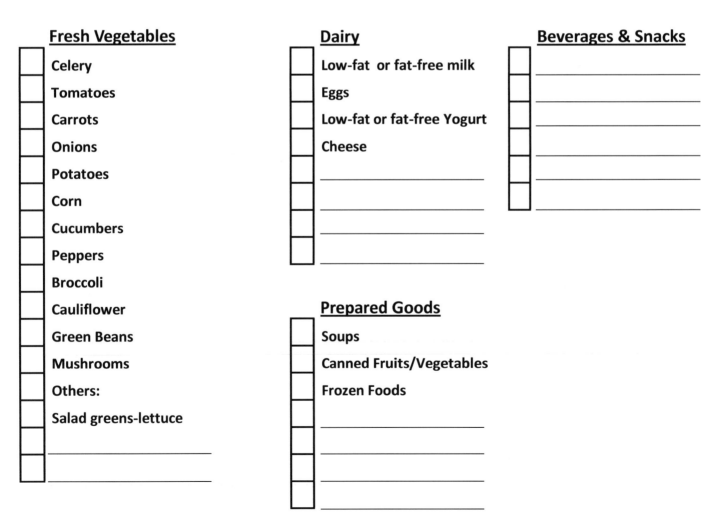

Fresh Vegetables

- [ ] Celery
- [ ] Tomatoes
- [ ] Carrots
- [ ] Onions
- [ ] Potatoes
- [ ] Corn
- [ ] Cucumbers
- [ ] Peppers
- [ ] Broccoli
- [ ] Cauliflower
- [ ] Green Beans
- [ ] Mushrooms
- [ ] Others:
- [ ] Salad greens-lettuce
- [ ] _____

Dairy

- [ ] Low-fat or fat-free milk
- [ ] Eggs
- [ ] Low-fat or fat-free Yogurt
- [ ] Cheese
- [ ] _____
- [ ] _____
- [ ] _____
- [ ] _____

Prepared Goods

- [ ] Soups
- [ ] Canned Fruits/Vegetables
- [ ] Frozen Foods
- [ ] _____
- [ ] _____
- [ ] _____

Beverages & Snacks

- [ ] _____
- [ ] _____
- [ ] _____
- [ ] _____
- [ ] _____
- [ ] _____

Choose 100% whole grains when available

FARMERS MARKET

Markets and community gardens are popping up all over, and we couldn't be more pleased. The trend to buy locally grown produce and foods is one many embrace but is certainly not new. Eleanor Roosevelt initiated the Community Gardens known as the *Victory Gardens of World War II*. Over 20 million gardens were planted and could be found on rooftops, in local parks, and private residences. Much like today, these markets supplied fresh foods, boosted moral, and connected people to each other and the land. Now, decades later, both city and rural areas offer Community Gardens. All that is required is a plot of land and a group of individuals with an interest in fresh, home grown foods.

Farmers markets, on the other hand, are found at only certain locations within a community. They are often in cities and offer a variety of fresh produce, foods, and flowers brought in by local farmers.

According to the U. S. Department of Agriculture (USDA), in 2009 there were 5,274 farmers markets in the U.S., a 42% increase from the previous 5 years and an 84% increase since 2000. Some are seasonal, some year-around. For those of us who enjoy experiencing new foods and tasting, smelling, and touching our foods, farmers markets are a joy.

Need one more reason to plant and pick your own foods?

According to the USDA, these are some of the advantages to shopping at farmers markets

- Enables growers and producers to develop personal relationships with customers
- Improves access to locally grown fresh produce
- Increases produce variety

10 Tips to get the most out of Famers Market shopping
(www.FruitandVeggieGuru.com)

- Make sure all vendors are growers/producers
- Shop early in the day for the best choices
- Shop seasonally
- Be prepared to spend more money for the value of some items
- Discover items not found at the local grocery store
- Ask how the foods were grown and processed
- Find out when the food was harvested
- Carry cash and a reusable shopping bag
- Get to know the seller/farmer

The American Journal of Public Health (June 2011) reported: More than half of those individuals who participated in community gardens met the nutrition recommendations to eat fruit and vegetables at least 5 times a day, compared to 37 percent of home gardeners and 25 percent of non-gardeners.

Find a location near your home and enjoy the fresh, unprocessed foods of the lands which you will be pleased to know are not too far away.
(See websites below)
- www.localharvest.org
- www.ams.usda.gov/farmersmarkets
- www.epicurious.com
- www.pickyourown.org

FOOD LABELS: NUTRITION AT A GLANCE

"TELL ME WHAT YOU EAT. I'LL TELL YOU WHO YOU ARE."
- JEAN ANTHELME BRILLAT, SAVARIN FRENCH LAWYER, POLITICIAN, EPICURE, AND GASTRONOME

Though food labels can be tricky to navigate, they are a wealth of information. To make the best possible food choices, you can't afford not to take a few seconds when shopping to read the nutrition label. Make sure to read the fine print and don't be swayed by the bold claims on the front of the package.

Food labels provide the necessary nutrient information for people following a special diet, looking to increase a particular nutrient, or just trying to eat healthy. On January 1, 2006, a new food label law called the Food Allergen Labeling and Consumer Protection Act of 2004 (FALCPA) went into effect. The law now requires manufactures to identify on the label if a product has any ingredients that contain protein derived from any of the eight major allergenic foods and food groups. These foods include: milk, eggs, fish, Crustacean shellfish, tree nuts, peanuts, wheat, or soybean. About 90 percent of all food allergies are related to these foods and food groups. FALCPA also requires the type of tree nut (e.g., almonds, pecans, walnuts); fish (e.g., bass, flounder, cod); and the type of Crustacean shellfish (e.g., crab, lobster, shrimp) to be listed.

A recent report from NPD Group's Dieting Monitor states that Americans are most interested in increasing the following: whole grains, dietary fiber, calcium, vitamin C, and protein. For most Americans, increasing protein isn't a concern, because on average, we already exceed our requirement. Iron, however, is often deficient in the diet particularly in adolescents and premenopausal women.

For those watching their weight or paying attention to sodium, fat and cholesterol, and calories, reading the food label is critical. No matter what the reason, healthy eating for many is dependent on understanding and interpreting a food label.

The sample food label below is for a packaged macaroni and cheese food product (label information taken from www.fda.gov/Food/ Labeling Nutrition). Let's take a look at the label. There are two parts to a food label:

Top section (1-4): has product-specific information such as serving size, calorie content, and nutrient information. This information varies with each food. On larger packages there is a footnote that provides information about important nutrients in that food.

Bottom section (5): the second part of the label has % daily values.

Nutrition Facts Label Design

1. Serving Size - Serving size reflects an individual portion size of the food item. All the nutrition information that follows on the label is based on this portion size. Serving sizes are generally provided in usual household measurements (e.g., cup), followed by the metric amount (e.g., grams). Remember, when you increase the portion size, you also increase the amount of calories and nutrients you are getting, and the % daily values. When watching

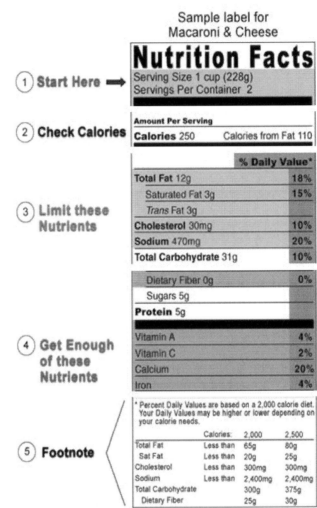

Sample label for Macaroni & Cheese

① Start Here ➡
② Check Calories
③ Limit these Nutrients
④ Get Enough of these Nutrients
⑤ Footnote

calories, it is important that you measure portions. The calories provided are for a single serving. Double the serving and you double the calories.

2. Calories — Besides telling you total calories per serving, the calories section on the label also tells you how many of the calories per serving come from fat. At a glance this information gives you an idea if the product is high in fat. For example, on our sample food label, a 1-cup serving of macaroni and cheese contains 250 calories and 110 calories from fat.   If you eat 2 cups of macaroni and cheese instead of only 1 cup, you may wind up taking in more calories from fat than what you had planned for the day.

3&4. Nutrients – This section identifies nutrients you may want to limit, followed by nutrients that Americans often don't get in adequate amounts. They are fiber, vitamin A, vitamin C, calcium, and iron. Fiber, in particular, is low in the average American diet. Taking the time to read and compare the food labels of breads and cereals, for example, can make it easy to increase your fiber intake.

% Daily Value * Column - The % Daily Value information makes it easy to compare one product's nutrition content to another. The % DVs is based on the recommended amounts of each nutrient for a 2,000 calorie/day diet. This information makes you aware of foods containing nutrients you might want to avoid or increase.   Most importantly, the % DV can help you determine if you are meeting the daily requirement of a nutrient. The rule of thumb for understanding % DV is if a serving has:

✓ Low in a nutrient = 5% DV or less of that nutrient

✓ Good Source of a nutrient = 10 to 19% DV of that nutrient

✓ High in a nutrient = 20% or more of that nutrient

5. Footnote - Last, but not least, on the nutrition panel is an asterisk (*), telling you the % DVs, shown in item 3 & 4, are based on a 2,000 calorie/day diet. Following this statement is nutritional information based on a 2,000 calorie and a 2,500 calorie a day diet. For example, on our sample food label, the recommendation for total fat, saturated fat, carbohydrate, and fiber is based on both a 2,000 calorie and a 2,500 calorie meal plan. Notice the recommendation for sodium and cholesterol is the same for all Americans and is not based on total calories.

For example, on our macaroni and cheese label, the product contains 20% of the calcium you need each day. In other words, if you eat 1 cup of macaroni and cheese, you have taken in about one-fifth of your day's requirement. If you add a glass of milk to this meal, you will have met more than half (50%) of your calcium needs for the day.

When shopping you may find yourself making decisions on what to purchase based on this nutrition information. The % Daily Value is a great guide that allows you to easily assess how nutritious a food is and how it fits into your healthy meal plan.

Currently, there are no % DVs for trans fat, sugar, or protein. Trans fat has been linked to heart disease, requiring manufacturers to begin listing trans fat on the nutrition panel beginning in January 2006. Companies can label foods as having no trans fat if the product has less than 0.5 grams of trans fats in a serving. But if you eat several servings of that product, trans fat can add up quickly. The American Heart Association recommends less than 2 grams trans fat per day. Make sure you take a look at the ingredients as well; if a food contains partially hydrogenated oils, it has trans fats. The label will not contain % DV for trans fat since medical experts have not yet determined what amount (if any) is safe.

Popular Product Label Terms: The front of the package can be confusing and misleading	
Food Processing Claims	
Natural	FDA's 1993 policy defines this term as not containing added color, artificial flavors, or synthetic substances. Use of this term is not permitted in the ingredient list, with the exception of the phrase "natural flavorings."
Processed vs. Unprocessed	The Farm Bill of 2008 states a processed food is a food that undergoes a "change of character."
Whole Food	Foods that are not processed or refined and do not have ingredients added to them are often labeled whole foods.
Organic Food	USDA states that organic foods including meat, poultry, eggs, and dairy come from animals that are given no antibiotics or growth hormones.
Health Claims	
Heart Healthy	Low in saturated fat, cholesterol, sodium, and has no trans fats.
Calories	
Light	Contains a third fewer calories than its full-calorie alternative.

Popular Product Label Terms: The front of the package can be confusing and misleading	
Calorie Free	Less than 5 calories per serving.
Low Calorie	Contains 40 calories or less per serving.
Carbohydrates	
Low Carb	Meaningless term, there's no definition for this term.
Sugar	
Sugar Free	Less than 0.5 grams of sugar per serving.
Reduced Sugar	At least 25% less sugar than the regular version.
Fiber	
High Fiber	Contains 5 g or more of fiber per serving.
Good Source of Fiber	2.5 g to 4.9 g of fiber per serving.
Sodium	
Sodium Free or Salt Free	Less than 5 mg of sodium per serving.
Very Low Sodium	35 mg of sodium or less.
Low Sodium	140 mg of sodium or less.
Reduced or Less Sodium	At least 25% less sodium than the regular version.
Fat	
Fat Free	Contains less than 0.5 gram of fat per serving.
Saturated Fat Free	Less than 0.5 g of saturated fat.
Low fat	Contains 3 g or less of total fat.
Low saturated fat	Has 1 g or less of saturated fat.
Reduced Fat or Less Fat	At least 25% less fat than the regular version.
No Trans Fat	Less than 0.5 g of trans fats.

Popular Product Label Terms: The front of the package can be confusing and misleading	
Cholesterol	
Cholesterol Free	Less than 2 mg per serving.
Low Cholesterol	Contains 20 mg or less cholesterol.
Reduced or Less Cholesterol	At least 25% less cholesterol than its original version.
Expiration Dates	
Sell-by	Tells the store how long to display the item. Purchase the product before the date expires.
Best if Used By (or Before)	Recommended for best flavor or quality. It is not a purchase-by or safety date.
Use-By	Dates reflect the last date recommended for the use of the product while at peak quality-determined by the manufacturer.

FDA allows precise health claims on the following:

- Calcium and Vitamin D (as of 2007) and osteoporosis

- Fat and Cancer

- Saturated Fat and Cholesterol and Coronary Heart Disease

- Fiber containing grain products, fruits, and vegetables and cancer

- Sodium and hypertension

- Fruits and vegetables and cancer

- Folic acid and neural tube defects

- Dietary sugar, alcohols, and dental caries

- Soluble fiber from certain foods and Coronary Heart Disease

You will find a % DV listed for protein only if a claim such as "high in protein" is made for a product. Unless the product is intended for use by infants and children under 4 years of age, a % DV for protein is not required. Protein is not considered to be a public health concern for adults and children over 4 years of age.

Lastly, there is no current recommendation for sugar in the diet. Sugar listed on the nutrition panel includes naturally occurring sugars like those found in milk and fruit, as well as added sugars, including high fructose corn syrup.

Though food manufactures may use health claims to market their products, the intended use is to make consumers aware of healthful eating patterns that may reduce the risk of heart disease, cancer, osteoporosis, high blood pressure, dental cavities, and some birth defects.

Over the years food labels have become food commercials. It is reassuring to know that the U.S. Food and Drug Administration is taking a look at food labels hoping to minimize the confusion related to all the health claims on food packages that currently exist. Until then, it's a good idea to be familiar with the terminology and remember that if it sounds too good to be true, it probably is.

EASY DINNERS

Coming home from work or a busy afternoon carpooling should not eliminate the possibility of putting a home cooked meal on the table. Planning out your menus in advance makes it possible to do some of the work ahead of time. This will enable you to cut down meal preparation when you hit the door.

Time how long it takes you to make a stop at a take-out or fast-food restaurant. Then time how long it takes you to put something easy together. Browning meat can be done the night before when you are washing dishes or in the morning when making lunches. When you have food available for leftovers, cut up the meat and decide how you will use it for another meal.

A great app that can help you plan easy dinners is named *The Healthy Gourmet: Inspired Eats.* This app is currently available through Apple's App Store and puts hundreds of recipes at the tip of your fingers.

The following pages are just a few ideas for quick and easy meals:

Quick Meal Entrée Ideas	Directions:
Spaghetti with lean beef/ turkey/ or marinara sauce	Put ground beef or ground turkey in a microwave safe baking dish. Break up into small pieces. Microwave until brown. Take out and drain off fat. Add water and drain. Pat dry. Add tomato sauce and microwave until warm.
Lean hamburgers or turkey burgers on a bun	Throw lean hamburgers in a frying pan or grill and brown.
Grilled tuna sandwich on a bun or English muffin	Mix one 5 ounce can of tuna with mayo. Top with a slice of 2% fat cheese. (makes two servings)

Quick Meal Entrée Ideas	Directions:
Beef, chicken, pork, fish, or bean fajitas	Cook peppers and onions in a skillet with olive oil or cooking sprays. Add to cooked beef, pork, fish or warmed up beans. Add 2% fat grated cheese and place on a tortilla.
Chicken, beef, fish or bean tacos	Add cooked chicken, beef, fish, or beans to a soft or hard tortilla. Add grated 2% cheese.
Kraft Macaroni and Cheese Casserole (mostly for the kids!)	Add lean cooked ground meat or turkey meat, ham chunks, chicken, or tuna. Add low sodium canned vegetables, or prepare fresh or frozen. Follow directions on package, use lite margarine and skim milk to reduce calories. Combine ingredients in a casserole. Sprinkle the top with bread crumbs. Bake in the oven for 20 minutes to combine flavors.
Barbequed pork on a light hamburger bun	If you have cooked a lean pork loin on the grill and have leftovers: Add barbeque sauce and a little water and cook until warm. Place on a hamburger bun.
Grilled Vegetables	Wash zucchini, eggplant, and/or carrots. Slice them large enough, through the width, so that they won't fall through the grill rack. Brush or drizzle with olive oil. Let each slice brown then remove them from the rack. Cut to desired serving size, or dice and add them to couscous or brown rice.
Cottage cheese and fruit and a large roll	Put ½ c. low-fat cottage cheese and fruit in a bowl. Add a large roll on the side.
Grilled beef, chicken, turkey, ham, pork, or lamb	Add any of these meats to grill. Cook until meat is cooked to preferred doneness. Add some grilled vegetables for a complete meal.
Grilled cheese sandwich (2% fat cheese) and cup of soup	Add low-fat margarine to two slices of bread. Add cheese and place in frying pan. Brown on one side and then the other. Open up a can of soup and warm or add a homemade soup made in advance.
Hot turkey/beef sandwich with low fat gravy	Warm up turkey or beef leftovers or buy turkey or beef at the deli counter. Warm with low-fat gravy. Place turkey or beef on sandwich bread with hot gravy.
Chili	Follow directions for spaghetti and meat sauce. Add 8 ounces of tomato sauce and a 26 ounce can of stewed tomatoes to the browned meat. Add 4 cans of kidney beans drained, a large cut up green pepper, a medium cut up onion, and 3 tbs. of chili powder. Cook in a slow cooker on either high or low depending on your needs.

Quick Meal Entrée Ideas	Directions:
Chili macaroni	Add ½ cup of cooked macaroni to a ½ cup of warmed chili.
Chicken, ham, tuna, roast beef or turkey roll-up	Place leftover cooked chicken, ham, turkey, or roast beef in roll-up. Or add tuna salad to the tortilla. See Roll-up meals for suggestions for what to add.
Bean, rice, and 2% cheese roll-up	Drain beans from can and warm in the microwave oven. Cook rice until done. Add grated 2% fat cheese. Roll ingredients in a tortilla. Try higher fiber tortillas for reduced calories.
Stuffed baked potato with 2% cheese and broccoli	Wash a potato. Poke with holes. Put a wet paper towel around the potato and place in microwave at microwave timing. Cook broccoli in microwave until cooked. Place 2% cheese on top of cooked baked potato and cook for 45 seconds. Top with hot broccoli.
Frozen pizza	Place in oven at recommended time.
Frozen ravioli with meat sauce	Boil ravioli for required time on package. Add meat sauce following spaghetti and meat sauce directions.
Sloppy Joe	Brown lean ground beef or ground turkey. Add tomato sauce and catsup to taste. Add chopped onion and green pepper.

Low Fat White Sauce

Ingredients
1 tbs. margarine
2 small cloves garlic, minced
1 1/3 cups skim milk
2 tbs. lite cream cheese
1 cup freshly grated Parmesan cheese
2 tsp. fresh parsley

Each serving equals:
5 grams Carbohydrate
11.7 grams Protein
12 grams Fat
175 calories

Melt margarine in a saucepan over medium heat. Add garlic and sauté for 1 minute. Stir in the flour and gradually add milk stirring with a wire whisk until it is blended. Cook approximately 8 minutes until thickened and bubbly stirring constantly. Add cream cheese and cook for 2 minutes. Add 1 cup of Parmesan cheese, stirring constantly, until melted. Add parsley. Makes 4 servings.

Pasta Dinners

Combine the items under the following categories to give you various pasta dinners

Pasta/Starch
- Whole wheat pasta any type (spaghetti, linguini, penne, ziti, etc)
- White pasta any type(spaghetti, linguini, penne, ziti, etc)
- Angel hair pasta cooks fast- approximately 3-5 minutes

Protein
- Grilled chicken breast
- Ground turkey/beef
- Beef/pork chunks
- Grilled salmon
- Shrimp/scallops/mussels/clams
- Turkey/chicken sausage
- Smart Ground –soy meat substitute
- Imitation crab-meat

Veggies
- Tomatoes
- Zucchini
- Eggplant
- Edamame
- Broccoli
- Mushrooms
- Spinach
- Sundried tomatoes
- Cauliflower

Sauces
- Marinara
- White wine
- Pesto
- Italian dressing
- Garlic/butter
- White sauce

Add-ins
- Bread crumbs
- Low-fat grated cheese

Spices
- Cloves
- Cinnamon sticks
- Olive oil
- Crushed red-pepper
- Garlic powder
- White wine

Roll-ups/ Wraps

Proteins
- Chicken
- Lean Beef
- Shrimp
- Salmon
- Tuna
- Imitation Crab
- Pork
- Grated Cheese (can be used alone or as a topping for the other proteins)
- Beans

Wraps/Tortillas
- Spinach
- Flour
- Wheat
- Black Bean

Fillers
- Lettuce
- Spinach
- Sugar snap peas
- Fresh cilantro
- Shredded carrots
- Cabbage
- Raisins
- Cranberries
- Mushrooms
- Black olives
- Tomato

Spreads
- Light mayo
- Honey Dijon
- Spicy brown mustard
- Yellow mustard
- Hummus
- Light cream cheese
- Avocado
- Salsa
- Light Italian Dressing

Stir-Fry Sauces

Getting Started

1. Heat your wok or skillet over low heat.
2. Marinate your protein choice in 1 tbsp. soy sauce and 1 tbsp. dry or sweet sherry. This can be done while cutting the produce chosen.
3. Cut produce.
4. Mince 1 tbsp. of garlic and ginger root.
5. Mix 2 tsp. cornstarch and 2 tbs. chicken broth or water.
6. Spray skillet or wok with Cooking Spray.
7. Stir-fry your protein choice until brown.
8. Add minced garlic and ginger root.
9. Add protein to wok or skillet.
10. Coat with any of the below sauces.
11. Stir in cornstarch mixture until juices are saucy and glossy. If the sauce appears too thick, add more chicken broth or water.
12. Serve the protein, produce, and sauce with rice, noodles, pasta, or couscous.

Fresh Cilantro Stir-Fry Sauce

Ingredients:
- ¼ cup chicken broth
- ¼ cup soy sauce
- 2 tsp. rice wine vinegar
- ½ tsp. sugar or 1 tsp artificial sweetener
- ¼ cup minced cilantro leaves

Mix together ingredients in a 1-cup measuring cup and pour over stir-fry mixture stirring frequently.
Calories are negligible for each serving. Makes 4 servings.

Sweet and Sour Stir-Fry Sauce

Ingredients:
- ¼ cup chicken broth
- 2 tbs. soy sauce
- 2 tbs. rice wine vinegar
- 1 tbs. brown sugar
- ½ tsp. hot red pepper flakes

Mix ingredients together in a 1-cup measuring cup and pour over stir-fry mixture stirring
frequently. Contains approximately 12 calories and 3 grams of carbohydrate for each serving.
Makes 4 servings.

Lemon Stir-Fry Sauce

Ingredients:
- ¼ cup chicken broth
- ¼ cup lemon juice
- 1 tsp. lemon zest
- 2 tbs. sugar or 2 tbs. sugar substitute
- 2 tbs. soy sauce

Mix together ingredients together in a 1-cup measuring cup. Pour over stir-fry mixture stirring frequently. Contains approximately 25 calories and 6 grams carbohydrate per serving. Using a sugar substitute in place of sugar reduces calories to negligible. Makes 4 servings.

Sesame Soy Sauce

Ingredients:
- ¼ cup chicken broth
- ¼ cup soy sauce
- 2 tsp. rice vinegar
- 1 tsp. red pepper flakes
- 1 tsp. sesame oil
- 1 tsp. sugar

Mix ingredients together in a 1-cup measuring cup. Pour over stir-fry mixture stirring frequently. Contains approximately 8 calories and 2 grams of carbohydrate per serving. Using a sugar substitute in place of sugar reduces the calories to negligible. Makes 4 servings.

Honey Soy Sauce

Ingredients:
- ¼ cup honey
- ½ cup rice vinegar
- 2 tbs. soy sauce
- 1 tbs. orange zest
- 1 tsp. red pepper flakes

Mix ingredients together in a 1-cup measuring cup. Pour over stir-fry mixture stirring frequently. Contains approximately 70 calories and 18 grams of carbohydrate per serving. Makes 4 servings.

Stir-Fry Combos

Stir-fry cooking can provide numerous quick meals. Mixing the groups below will provide many menu ideas.

Protein
- Chicken strips
- Shrimp
- Scallops
- Pork chunks
- Beef strips
- Tofu

Starch
- Wild rice
- White rice
- Rice Noodles
- Couscous
- Noodles
- Pasta
- Quinoa

Flavorings
- La Choy Soy sauce
- Sesame oil
- Garlic
- Ginger

Nuts
- Peanuts
- Cashews
- Almonds
- Walnuts

Vegetables
- Green, red, & yellow peppers
- Broccoli
- Sugar snap peas
- Asparagus
- Zucchini
- Mushrooms
- Celery
- Scallions
- Onions
- Frozen stir-fry vegetables

Directions
Cook rice or rice noodles. Add vegetable spray to skillet and add protein choice until thoroughly cooked. Remove protein from skillet and move to the side. Add vegetables to skillet cooking until tender for about 3-4 minutes. Put protein back into the skillet with vegetables and add flavorings, heating for 1 extra minute.

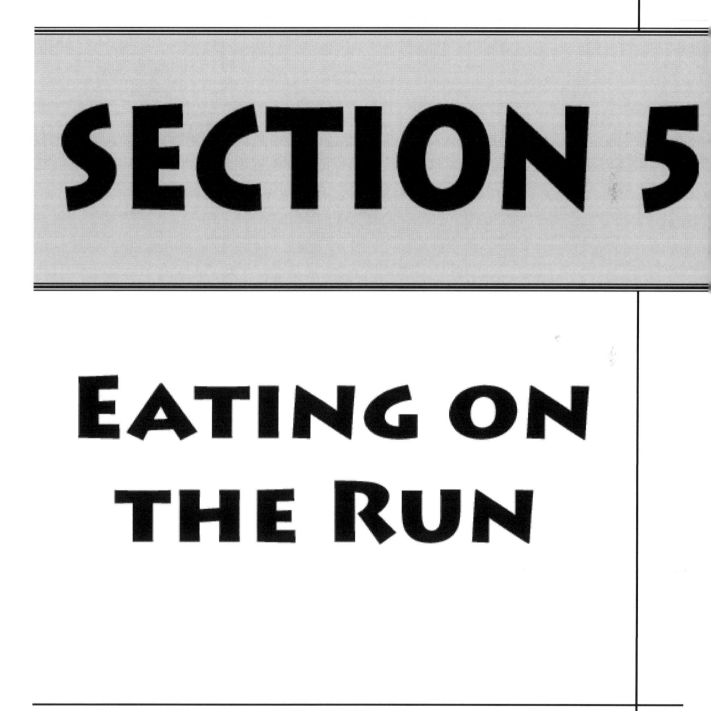

SECTION 5

EATING ON THE RUN

BREAKFAST

Starting the day with breakfast is smart. Breakfast is good for you and there are many good reasons to slow down and take the time to eat breakfast. Research has shown that breakfast is the most important meal of the day and when consumed, people generally make better food choices later in the day. Those that eat breakfast also tend to get more fiber, calcium, riboflavin, zinc, iron, and vitamins A and C, as well as less fat and cholesterol. The American Journal of Clinical Nutrition reported in 2010 that those that skipped breakfast throughout childhood and as adults had higher levels of LDL (bad cholesterol) than those that had always eaten breakfast. The good news is that there are many fast, easy, and nutritious foods available that make starting the day with breakfast a no-brainer.

REVVING YOUR ENGINE

Breakfast means literally "break the fast." When we wake up after a night's sleep, we are in a fasting state (or starvation mode). You can jump start your metabolism by eating something first thing in the morning. When we eat something we literally wake up the digestive system, stimulating our metabolism. Skipping breakfast causes individuals to remain in a fasting state resulting in slower metabolism and the potential to interfere with weight loss efforts.

Many people complain to us that they just aren't hungry in the morning. More often than not, they've eaten a late dinner or snacked at bedtime. By avoiding eating late at night you'll be more likely to wake up hungry and look forward to breakfast. If you just don't care to eat first thing in the morning, plan to have something one or two hours after you get up. If you are stopping at your favorite fast food restaurant, know that there are healthy breakfast choices such as an egg white English muffin sandwich, fruit smoothies, and low-fat yogurts with fresh fruit. Or alternatively, bring a lite morning snack to work like a piece of fruit with cheese, or crackers, or a yogurt with granola or nuts.

After years of working with overweight patients, we have found that individuals who skip breakfast tend to overeat later in the day. They also tend to select foods higher in sugar and fat. When people select high-fiber breakfast foods, they typically find themselves feeling less hungry during the day and later evening. As a result, there is an overall lower caloric consumption and a spreading out of calories throughout the day which has been shown to be healthier for the body and soul.

Research has also found that eating breakfast can improve school and work performance. Eating breakfast can aid with the following:

- Help with problem-solving, alertness, memory, and learning

- Increase scores on creativity tests

- Enhance alertness, which helps with memory and learning

- Allow attentiveness, retention of material, and increased interest in learning new things

- Improve mood, increase calmness, and reduce stress

Interestingly, an increased carbohydrate intake is associated with improved mood. The B vitamins, folate, and thiamin, have also been found to improve mood, and thiamin has been found to increase feelings of well-being. For all of these reasons, it is important to incorporate eating breakfast into your busy day.

BREAKFAST TIPS

Breakfast can be easily packed with nutrition by discovering a few healthy items that are easy to prepare and that you enjoy. It is also one of the quickest and easiest meals to put together since many breakfast foods do not require cooking. Make sure you include protein in your meal. Aim for at least 5 grams of protein for a balance of nutrients and to prevent those feelings of hunger that can appear two to three hours after an all carbohydrate meal. A breakfast with some protein and high quality carbohydrates that have fiber can aid in weight loss efforts by keeping you feeling fuller longer.

Scramble some egg whites or egg beaters and sandwich them between some whole grain toast or an English muffin. Don't forget that an 8 oz. glass of orange juice fortified with calcium and vitamin D will provide 120% of your vitamin C, 35% of your calcium, and 25% of your vitamin D daily requirements.

You can drink your breakfast by making a fruit smoothie, combining low fat milk or yogurt and fresh fruit, or drinking an already prepared beverage. You can add protein powder to a beverage for added protein. Here are some suggestions for easy nutritious breakfasts:

- Top breakfast cereals with fresh, frozen, canned, or dried fruits: pineapple, bananas, berries, raisins, cranberries, dates, or apricots.

- Mix a variety of breakfast cereals together to give a mixture of tastes and textures. Look for high fiber breakfast cereals. At least 5 grams.

- Add nuts to cereal (hot or cold for a crunchy taste).

- For a taste of sweetness, try a teaspoon of chocolate chips or five mini-marshmallows.

- Add low-fat granola or nuts to your low fat yogurt.

- Hard boiled eggs

- Peanut butter on an apple (refrigerate for a few minutes)

- Many people forget that vegetables can also be added to breakfast. Drink a glass of tomato juice or load your omelet with tomatoes, spinach, or both.

Try some non-traditional types of food for breakfast such as the following:

- Grilled cheese (and tomato) sandwich, peanut butter and banana sandwich, peanut butter on raisin toast or whole grain bread, cottage cheese or plain yogurt with fresh or canned fruit, hard cooked eggs, or mozzarella sticks.

- Breakfast pizza or Hawaiian breakfast pizza.

- Try some typical dessert items such as rice pudding with a reduced amount of sugar.

- Cheese chunks with fresh fruit such as grapes or apple slices.

- Make your own breakfast cereal bars.

- Whole wheat English muffins with cheese, peanut butter, or Canadian bacon

- Glucerna Bars

- Glucerna Shakes

- Carnation Instant Breakfast

- Slim-Fast shakes

- Nutrition bars (see Chapter 35)

CHOOSING BREAKFAST CEREALS

It is important to watch the sugar content of cereals selected. Manufacturers of breakfast cereals pay a lot of money to obtain grocery store shelf space that will enhance your choice of particular types of cereals. Sugary cereals are generally at shopping cart level where children will see them and attempt to convince their parents to purchase the cereals advertised during the Saturday morning cartoon's commercials. At the adult eye level, we find sweetened adult cereals that tempt us to make impulsive decisions. In general, the top shelf contains the healthier choices, along with those that boast of being healthier (but in reality are not).

To help you make the right decision for healthy cereals, focus on these key label items:

- serving size

- fiber

- calories

- carbohydrate and sugar content

The weight of a serving is generally 30 grams, but can vary from one-third to two cups depending on the cereal's fluffiness and packaging of the flakes. A good portion size for the average person is one and a half cups of cereal. Athletes will generally consume at least three cups of cereal at one time.

High fiber cereals are those that provide four grams of fiber per serving and very high fiber cereals contain six grams of fiber or more. Remember that you should consume 25- 40 grams of fiber each day.

A cereal's sugar content is very important when selecting a breakfast cereal. Check the label for the *total carbohydrate* content. Under this heading look for sugar. This is how much sugar (in grams) that is in one serving of your cereal. Every 4 grams of sugar on the label is the equivalent to adding a teaspoon of sugar to the cereal. If a cereal label states it contains 14 grams of sugar, that is the equivalent of 3 ½ teaspoons of sugar.

Dietitians and dentists recommend that you choose cereals that contain fewer than 6 grams of sugar per serving. Childhood obesity and tooth decay are two health risks that can be reduced with reduction of sugar intake. There are more than 40 breakfast cereals on the market that contain 6 grams of sugar or less. Government guidelines recommend that any cereal with sugar content greater than 10% of calories in a serving of the item is too high in sugar. For example, if a cereal contains 160 calories, it should not contain more than 16 calories or one teaspoon of sugar.

You can piece together a healthy, well-balanced breakfast that takes just a few minutes. Try and include at least two or three of the following: whole grains, low-fat dairy, protein and fruits when possible. We hope breakfast becomes a natural part of your day.

PLAN FOR PACKED MEALS

Whether you sit down for a hot breakfast or grab something on the run, having breakfast is a must. It helps get your metabolism running and prevents hunger later in the day. More important is its role in keeping you alert and on top of your game. Below is a list of foods that you can pack in a briefcase, diaper bag, or paper sack.

Bagged Breakfast Ideas:	
Fresh fruit	Hard Roll with All-fruit Jelly or Jam
Canned 100% Juice or 100% Juice Box	Low-Fat Yogurt
Granola Bar	Cheese and Crackers
Energy Bar	Peanut Butter and Crackers
Bagel	Peanut Butter and Apples
Low-Fat Muffins	Peanut Butter Sandwich
Bagel Chips	Mozzarella Cheese Sticks
Graham Crackers	Hard-Cooked egg
Dry Cereal (calcium fortified if possible)	Fruit or Applesauce Cups
Hot Cereal Packets (add hot water at the office)	Dried Fruit
	Nuts
Whole Wheat Bread	Healthy trail mix

When you are too busy to go out for lunch or dinner, bag lunches and dinners can be a smart idea. The advantage of bag meals is that you are controlling what you're eating and not worrying about what is added to the food. If you can bring a bag lunch or dinner to work, on the way to an appointment, or when running errands, your calories will be more easily managed. A bagged meal will be especially helpful if you are on the road and unfamiliar with local restaurants.

Bag lunches and dinners can get boring if the same sandwich is packed each day. Try adding variety by varying the type of sandwich fillings, breads, spreads, and sauces. If you have access to a microwave and refrigerator, a frozen lunch or dinner is a good option. Try adding a fruit, vegetable, and possibly a starch serving to frozen meals.

Varied Sandwich Ideas
Sliced cooked meats/cold cuts
Chicken
Lean corned beef
Lean ham
Lean roast beef
Turkey
Turkey pastrami
Turkey bologna
Turkey salami
Breads
Whole wheat
7 grain bread
Rye
Pumpernickel
Sour dough
Tortillas- Flour, Whole Wheat, Spinach, Sun-dried tomato
Pita bread- Regular, Whole wheat
Rolls
Bagels

Varied Sandwich Ideas

Eggs

Medium to Hard Poached
Scrambled
Hard-cooked

Fillers

Lettuce- try varying the type
Tomato
Red Onion
Avocado slices
Sauerkraut
Chopped apple
Chopped nuts
Olives
Bacon bits

Spreads

Regular and lite mayonnaise
Flavored mayonnaise, e.g., chipotle
Dijonnaise
Barbeque sauce
Mustard
Honey mustard
Catsup
Chili sauce
Sour cream lite or regular
Horseradish sauce

Reduced Fat Cheeses

Cheddar
Colby
Cream Cheese
Swiss
Processed cheese

Sandwich Salads (Low Fat Mayonnaise Options)

Chicken
Corned beef
Crabmeat
Egg
Salmon
Shrimp
Tuna
Turkey

THE SKINNY ON SNACKS

Call it what you like: snacking, grazing, noshing; we are a snacking society. There is probably no other country that snacks throughout the day as much as we do. Offices and homes are small convenience stores, making it difficult to avoid the temptation to snack. Some individuals admit to snacking because of boredom or merely because snacks are available, rather than snacking from hunger. For others, snacks are a reward for a tough or busy day at work or dealing with a grouchy boss. One of the drawbacks to frequent snacking is that we tend to forget what it's like to feel hunger. The end result is that we wind up never feeling satisfied and eating too many calories.

Not to worry. Snacks can be a great opportunity for some quick nutrition, a pick me up during the day, or even a little guilty pleasure. If you're trying to lose weight, snacks prevent overeating at the next meal, especially if the meal is delayed.

✓ **Think before you snack.** Snacking is often impulsive. And visual cues can be the strongest, tempting us to eat even if not hungry. Ask yourself: am I really hungry; when's my next meal; is there an activity I can do instead of eating? Remember a bite here and there eventually adds up.

✓ **Do the math.** Know the calories in the snack you choose, and make sure it fits into your meal plan. Regardless of the nutritional value of a snack, those snack calories are included in your calorie budget. When you exceed your daily allowance, you will gain weight. In fact, if you add 100 calories a day to your current intake with no changes to your activity, you can gain

10 lbs. in one year. It doesn't matter if the snack is an apple or a small Snickers bar. Those extra calories will catch up with you, usually around your waistline.

✓ **Limit your choices.** Select a few snacks you enjoy and are within your calorie budget. There's a large variety of snack items to choose from. Many are available in 100 calorie packs. Even Twinkies has joined the 100 calorie snack packs. Baggie your favorites: baby carrots, nuts, dried fruit, pretzels, dark chocolate. Planning ahead and allowing for snacks based on their calories and nutrition is the smart way to go.

✓ **Kitchen is Closed!** Night snacking can pack on the pounds. Most of us eat enough dinner to avoid eating again. There's not much time until bed, so we don't work off those extra calories. If you really want something, try a low calorie beverage or snack. Keep in mind that snacking will make you stay up longer. If you are tired, go to sleep.

Low carbohydrate, high fiber snacks are a good idea since they will make you feel fuller longer without the extra calories. Fruits and vegetables are good choices. If there is a long time between meals, say more than five hours, a snack with a little protein or fat is a better choice. Fat and protein will stay with you longer, getting you from meal to meal with a minimal amount of hunger. You will then be able to avoid overeating at that next meal.

Avoid using beverages as snacks. Liquids usually don't keep you satisfied for long; you'll find yourself looking for something else to eat an hour or two later. Juices provide very little nutrition and often contain a lot of sugary calories. Read the label before you drink.

Remember snacking can be nutritious and easy to incorporate into a healthy eating plan.

SNACKING ON THE GO

For busy people on the go, it's easy to skip meals without ever realizing a meal was missed. You may be caught in a meeting, rushing to make a deadline, or running to drop kids off at school. Despite a hectic schedule, it is important to allow yourself something to eat every four to five hours. This will help avoid feelings of extreme hunger that lead to overeating and weight gain.

If there is a refrigerator at work or school, keep a supply of bottled water, diet pop, yogurt, cheese, frozen meals, and fruit on hand. A microwave will allow a quick warm up of leftovers, frozen meals, canned soups, popcorn, and hot cereal. Thinking through food needs will avoid visits to the vending machine or take-out restaurants, where choices are high in calories, fat, and cholesterol.

The same holds true when traveling from place to place in the car: keep a supply of healthy snack foods on hand when stopping for a meal isn't possible. A collapsible cooler will provide a cool spot to keep beverages and food safe while traveling. A sport cooler can be purchased at sporting good stores, Target, or Wal-Mart. They are great for individuals who travel for work. Slip the cooler into a side pocket of a suitcase for use in the hotel room.

When traveling by plane for business or pleasure, make sure to bring a carry-on bag for snacks. As a result of current security measures, most airlines suggest not packing food in suitcases to be checked. Liquid items cannot be brought through the security check-in, but can be purchased once past security.

With today's airline travel, it's easy to get delayed in security checks that allow little time to stop for a meal. And, when there is time, the food is often full of calories and fat. Pre-planning carry-on food for the plane and hotel will eliminate the need for impulse eating. This type of eating is often the result of fatigue, fewer eating choices, and stress.

If renting a car, take advantage of the local grocery store rather than the high calorie foods from room service or lobby vending machines. A quick call to the hotel before leaving will provide helpful information about grocery or drug store accessibility, where food and beverages can be purchased for more individual needs.

SNACKS UNDER 50 CALORIES

CRUNCHY SNACKS

Food	Portion	Calories
Air-popped popcorn	1 cup	30
Dill pickle	1 medium	12
Melba Toast	2 pieces	25
Oyster Crackers	10	33
Saltine crackers	3	40

SWEET TREATS

Food	Portion	Calories
Creamsicle	1 low-cal	25
Meringue cookie	1 cookie	35
Flavored sugar free gelatin	1 cup	20
Unsweetened applesauce	½ cup	50
Chewing gum	1 stick	5
Fortune cookie	1	15
Gummy Bears	3	20
Hard candy	1 piece	25
Ice pop	2 fl. oz. bar	42
Life savers	4 pieces	36
Lollipop	1	22
Marshmallow	2 large	46
Whipped topping	2 tablespoons	25
Sugar-free jelly/jam	2 teaspoons	30

FABULOUS FRUIT

Food	Portion	Calories
Apricots	3 medium	50
Blackberries	½ cup	37
Cranberries	1 cup	46
Watermelon	½ cup	30
Apple	1 small	50
Water packed fruit cocktail	½ cup	40
Grapefruit	½ medium	37
Orange	1 small	50
Kiwi	1 medium	46
Peach	1 medium	37
Fresh mixed fruit	1 cup	50
Grapes	15	50
Cherries	12	50
Strawberries	1 cup	50
Banana	½	40

SNACKS UNDER 100 CALORIES

GREAT GRAINS

Food	Portion	Calories
Raisin bread	1 slice	60
Whole wheat bread	1 slice	70
Rye bread	1 slice	70
Plain bagel	½ medium	88

HOW CHEESY

Food	Portion	Calories
Low-fat string cheese	1 piece	80
Low-fat cottage cheese	½ cup	90

PORTABLE FRUITS

Food	Portion	Calories
Banana	½	53
Blueberries	1 cup	82
Cantaloupe	1 cup cubed	57
Fruit salad	½ cup	67
Grapes	1 cup	58
Honeydew melon	1 cup cubed	60
Mango	½ medium	68
Nectarine	1 medium	67
Orange	1 medium	65
Papaya	½ medium	58

HOT, HOT, HOT

Food	Portion	Calories
Vegetable soup	1 cup	72
Chicken noodle soup	1 cup	75
Baked crab cakes	1 cake	88

SOMETHING SWEET: LIMIT THESE CHOICES

Food	Portion	Calories
Rice Krispies	1 bar	90
Special-K bar	1 bar	90
Snack Wells Crème sandwich	2 cookies	86
Snickers Snack size	1 snack size	52
Twix snack size	1 snack size	80
3 Musketeers snack size	3 snack size	75
Licorice	2 pieces	70
Reese's minis	2 mini cups	84
Candy corn	10 pieces	51
Sugar-free pudding	1 cup	92
Fig bar	1	53
Gingersnaps	2	59
Graham crackers	1 large square	60
Wafers- chocolate or vanilla	3	75
Animal crackers	5	56

KEEPIN' COOL

Food	Portion	Calories
Fat-free fudgsicle	1 bar	60
Fat-free frozen yogurt	½ cup	70
Italian chocolate ice	1 scoop	60
Fruit sorbet	1 scoop	60
Fat-free ice cream	½ cup	90
Frozen fruit and juice bar	1 bar	75

MUNCH ON THIS....

Food	Portion	Calories
Baked Chips	11 chips	110
Baked Tortilla Chips	20 chips	110
Soy Chips	25 chips	110
Triscuits	7	120
Sun Chips	10 chips	140
Pretzel Rods	3 rods	110
Veggie Crisps	21 crisps	140
Mini Rice Cakes	15	120
Wheat Thins	16	150
English Muffin	1	126

SWEET TREATS

Food	Portion	Calories
Chex Morning Mix	1 pkg.	130
Quaker Chewy Granola Bar	1 bar	110
Hot Chocolate	1 pkg.	150
Angel Food Cake	1 slice	145
Jelly Beans	10	104
Italian Ice	½ cup	120

SNACKS UNDER 200 CALORIES

GO NUTS!

Food	Portion	Calories
Almonds	1 oz	166
Cashews	1 oz	170
Pecans	1 oz	186
Peanuts	1 oz	160
Pumpkin seeds	¼ cup	160
Sunflower seeds	2/3 cup	170
Walnuts	1 oz	172

THE OTHER STUFF

Food	Portion	Calories
Carnation Instant Breakfast	1 pkg.	200
Tuna- water packed	1 can	191
Regular gelatin	1 cup	160
Trail mix	½ cup	173
Nature Valley granola bar	1 pkg. (2 bars)	200

MIX IT UP!

Food	Portion	Calorie Mix	Total Calories
Cottage cheese/Mixed fruit	½ cup/ 1 cup	100/50	150
Cheese/Crackers	1 oz/ 6 crackers	80/78	158
Peanut butter/Whole wheat bread	1 Tbsp/1 slice	78/60	138
Raisin bread/Sugar-free jelly	1 slice/2 tsp	60/50	110
Baked tortilla chips/Salsa	20 chips/ 6 Tbsp	110/ 45	155
Skim milk/Special K bar	½ cup/ 1 bar	45/90	135
Skim milk/Graham crackers	½ cup/ 2 lg square	45/120	165
Veggie soup/Oyster crackers	1 cup/ 10	72/33	105
Fat-free yogurt/Grape nuts cereal	8 oz/ 1 oz	50/100	150
Apple/Peanut butter	1 medium/ 1 Tbsp	60/87	147

Miscellaneous Snacks								
Item	Size	Calories	Carbohydrate (grams)	Protein (grams)	Fat (grams)	Cholesterol (mg)	Sodium (mg)	Fiber (grams)
Einstein Brownie	122 gm.	500	76	4	21	30	280	2
Einstein Chocolate Chip Cookie	113 gm.	600	78	4	28	45	480	2
Einstein Sugar Cookie	113 gm.	610	73	7	32	55	490	1
Einstein Banana nut muffin	142 gm.	520	59	9	29	95	430	3
Einstein Chocolate chip muffin	57 gm.	240	67	3	13	40	370	0
Einstein Cinnamon Bun with icing	113 gm.	380	64	8	10	0	310	2
Einstein Blueberry Scone	127 gm.	450	64	7	18	55	460	2
Einstein Low fat Raspberry Scone	117 gm.	350	74	7	3	25	330	2
Krispy Kreme Donut (glazed ring)	52 gm.	200	23	4	11	5	115	2

Miscellaneous Snacks Continued								
Item	Size	Calories	Carbohydrate (grams)	Protein (grams)	Fat (grams)	Cholesterol (mg)	Sodium (mg)	Fiber (grams)
Einstein Egg Bagel	69 gm.	340	69	11	3	35	510	2
Einstein Cinnamon Swirl Bagel	113 gm.	350	78	11	1	0	490	2
Einstein Power Bagel w/ peanut butter	117 gm.	750	92	27	34	0	780	7
Einstein Cranberry Bagel	113 gm.	350	78	10	1	0	490	3
Dunkin Donut Plain Croissant	NA	290	26	5	18	5	270	<1
Dunkin Donut Chocolate Chip Muffin	NA	590	88	9	24	75	560	3
Dunkin Donut Corn Muffin	NA	500	78	10	16	80	920	1
Dunkin Donut Lemon Poppyseed Muffin	NA	580	94	10	19	85	620	2

Miscellaneous Snacks Continued

Item	Size	Calories	Carbohydrate (grams)	Protein (grams)	Fat (grams)	Cholesterol (mg)	Sodium (mg)	Fiber (grams)
Dunkin Donut Chocolate Bismark Muffin	NA	340	50	3	15	0	290	<1
Dunkin Donut traditional	NA	240	25	3	15	0	340	<1
Krispy Kreme Chocolate Donut (Iced Glazed)	66 gm.	280	36	3	14	>5	75	1
Einstein Chocolate chip bagel	113 gm.	370	76	11	3	0	500	3

Sample Snack Recipe

Trail Mix:

1 cup wheat chex
1 cup rice chex
1 cup corn chex
1 cup raisins
1 cup dry roasted peanuts
Mix the above together in a large bowl. 3 cups of cheerios can be substituted for the chex; dried cranberries can be used in place of the raisins.

Makes 10 (1/2 cup) servings	Makes 15 (1/3 cup) servings
Each serving = 152 calories 25 grams Carbohydrate 4 grams Protein 5 grams Fat	Each serving= 100 calories 17 grams Carbohydrate 3 grams Protein 3 grams Fat

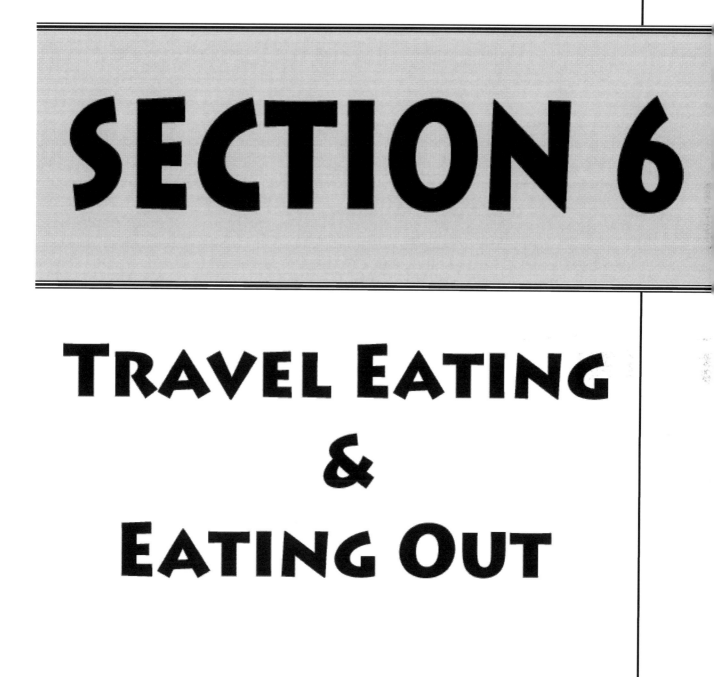

SECTION 6

TRAVEL EATING
&
EATING OUT

TRAVEL EATING

When a majority of time is spent in the car, running from appointment to appointment, it's helpful to have a method for eating on the road. Many sales representatives (and moms!) keep a basket of healthy snacks in the trunk that can be grabbed between appointments. Even if you're short on time, a healthier, and cheaper, food choice is as close as the trunk! Collapsible coolers are useful to store items such as diet cold drinks, water, yogurt, low-fat cheese, and sandwiches. Just stick a cold pack in the cooler to keep things cold. These can be purchased at Target, K-Mart, Wal-Mart, or sporting goods stores. The advantage of a collapsible cooler is that it takes up little space and can be folded in the outside pocket of a suitcase when traveling, in addition to use in the car. If traveling overnight, fill the cooler with ice if you do not have a refrigerator in your room.

Try to keep a source of protein available if you are unable to stop for a quick meal. This would include peanut butter or nuts if a cooler isn't available. With a cooler or refrigerator, foods can include:

- Yogurt
- Cheese, reduced fat
- Lunch meats, low-fat
- Bottled Water
- Juice Bottles or Boxes
- Fresh fruit or fruit cups

When staying at a hotel, try to book hotels that provide a breakfast buffet. These hotels typically offer eggs, bagels, toast, waffles, cereals, fresh fruit, yogurt, juice, and hot breakfast drinks. Take care when selecting food from the buffet, and think through your choices based upon your healthy meal plan. Sitting at a restaurant and ordering a meal will often encourage you to indulge in larger servings which include greater amounts of high calorie, high fat food.

FUELING AT THE GAS STATION

Hard to believe a couple of dietitians are recommending stopping at a gas station for a quick pick-me-up snack or meal? Suffice it to say that gas station foods have changed over the years. Chewing gum, candy bars, donuts, and sodas are still the first shelf when we walk in the door, but are no longer the only choices to pick from when hungry and on the road. Some gas stations have mini-markets offering a variety of foods and snacks. Grab a nutritious snack or piece together a few items to make a meal that fits into your healthy meal plan.

Here are a few healthy options that most gas stations carry	
cereal	granola bars
fat-free milk	deli sandwiches
fresh fruit	soups (broth-based)
cheese	nuts
whole grain crackers and breads	bottled water or flavored water

Use our list of healthy snacks and see what other items you might find when stopping to fuel up!

Gas station foods to avoid:	
regular soda	nachos
candies	hot dogs
sweetened coffee drinks	donuts and pastries
sweetened energy drinks	cookies and brownies
chips	

AIRPORT TRAVEL

Airline travel is a common part of a busy life. With the stress of post 9/11 and increased security, air travel has changed a great deal. Longer time is required at the airports to deal with security issues. Based upon recent cutbacks, domestic flights no longer offer meals in flight for most passengers. More individuals are eating at airports or buying food to eat on the plane.

Airports are beginning to respond to the public's desire for fast and easy meals and quick to grab beverages. Customers are also demanding healthier food choices to meet their nutritional needs. Today, 83% of the top U.S. airports have met the demand by acknowledging more than 50% of restaurants provide healthy choices. The fifteen busiest US airports are listed below with their scores for availability of healthy food choices. Scores were determined by the inclusion of at least one low-fat, high-fiber, and low cholesterol entrée. The final % score was determined by dividing the total number of restaurants offering a healthy entrée by the total number of restaurants.

Airport Score for Restaurants Offering Healthy Entrée's			
Detroit Metropolitan Wayne County	100%	Phoenix Sky Harbor	81%
San Francisco	96%	Charlotte Douglas	81%
Washington Dulles	71%	Orlando	80%
Minneapolis– St. Paul	86%	Los Angeles	76%
Dallas/Forth Worth	83%	Baltimore/Washington	76%
Las Vegas	83%	Ronald Reagan Washington	75%
Denvar	82%	Hartsfield-Jackson Atlanta	71%
Miami	82%		

Reprinted with Permission from the Physicians Committee for Responsible Medicine 2011

Whether traveling by car, or plane, there are some foods that provide good nutrition, moderate calories, and minimize hunger. Do check the TSA website for what foods are prohibited until after security check, such as beverages.

Travel Food List		
Bottled water	Bagels	Canned light sugar fruits
Diet pop	Whole grain cereal boxes	Peanut butter (except planes)
Juice boxes or juice cans	Low-fat popcorn bags	Nuts
Raisins	Pretzels	Low-fat cheeses
Dried fruits	Baked chips	Fresh Fruit
Healthy trail mixes	Low-fat cookies	Sandwiches
Whole grain crackers	Graham crackers	Rice cakes
100-calorie snack packs by Nabisco and Kraft	Nutrition Bars	Vegetables with low-fat dips

VENDING MACHINES

We've come a long way from the first vending machine recorded in 215 BCE, which dispensed holy water in Egyptian temples. The first vending machine to appear in the U.S. was in 1888 dispensing Tutti-Frutti gum in the subways of New York City. After years of same old/same old, vending machines are finally getting a high tech makeover. Kraft's and Coca-cola's new machines will resemble large iPhones. You'll be able to pick your product, enlarge it if necessary and even review the nutrition information. We're hoping that having access to nutrition information will translate into smart choices.

Vending machines are designed to tempt those who are hungry, un-prepared, and short on time. They can lure us with high calorie, high sugar, high sodium, and high fat choices. Most vending machine users have skipped a meal or find themselves in a situation where food isn't available. The following suggestions can help to reduce your calories from vending machines.

Tips for Reducing Calories from Vending Machines

Plan ahead: Make a list of healthy snacks that can be purchased at your grocery and can be stashed in your desk or office refrigerator.

• Bottled water	• Rice cakes	• Juice boxes
• Diet pop	• Whole grain cereal boxes	• Peanut butter
• Raisins	• Low-fat popcorn	• Nuts
• Dried fruits	• Graham crackers	• Low-fat cheese sticks
• Healthy trail mixes	• Low-fat cookies	• Fruits/Vegetables
• Whole grain crackers	• Canned no sugar fruits	• Low-Fat Yogurt

---

More Tips for Reducing Calories

<u>Label:</u>   Keep snacks in a baggie and label the calories to discourage food thieves.

<u>Prepare Choices:</u> Study the items found in the vending machine to find the healthy snacks and choose these snacks when the urge hits. This will reduce making impulsive choices.

<u>Rewards:</u> Compare the cost of the healthy choices from the vending machine with the cost of the same items purchased at the store. Put your savings into a jar and reward yourself periodically with special treats. Examples would include: having a Starbucks cappuccino with skim milk, and non-food treats such as movie tickets, manicure, or massage.

<u>Reduce Impulse Buying:</u> Limit the amount of change you keep in your pocket or desk drawer

Snack items selected should be counted as part of your overall daily meal plan. Rule of thumb: limit snacks to 150 calories for each snack and limit yourself to 2-3 snacks each day (depending on your personal nutrition plan).

> Limit snacks to 150 calories for each snack and limit yourself to 2-3 snacks each day.

Healthy Vending Machine Snacks	
Bottled water	Low fat popcorn
Diet pop	Nuts
100% fruit juice	Canned fruit
Dried fruit	Fresh fruit
Whole grain cereal bars	Turkey, ham, chicken sandwiches
Skim milk	Tea (unsweetened or diet)
Pretzels	Decaffeinated coffee plain

Unhealthy Vending Machine Snacks	
High fat cookies	Cheese
Candy	Sausage meats
Chips	Sandwich crackers
High fat crackers	Regular soda
Cakes	Regular punch or lemonade
Cupcakes	Whole milk

DINING OUT

Test your Dining Out knowledge by answering <u>True</u> or <u>False</u> to the following questions:

1. You cannot follow a healthy diet when you eat out.
2. Fast-foods can never be eaten if you are trying to lose weight.
3. Layering a meal with a variety of foods will only cause you to eat too many calories.
4. The average American eats out one or two times per week.
5. Alcohol can fill you up and diminish your appetite.

Let's face it. Eating out frequently means we increase our chances of eating more calories and gaining weight. Serving sizes in many restaurants are bigger than ever. Dinner plates, like portion sizes, have grown. What ever happened to the 8 inch dinner plate? The average dinner plate is now around 12 inches and chefs are happy to pile on the portions.

A study in the Journal of Obesity, 2007, reported when chefs were interviewed, they stated, "regular size" portions are served 76% of the time. In reality, "regular size" portions of steak and pasta are 2 to 4 times larger than the serving size recommended by the U.S. Government. Planning your meals in advance and establishing reliable strategies can help you make good choices and eat healthy while dining out.

Learn to navigate restaurant menus. Most restaurants will accommodate requests to order from the children's menu, split a meal, or choose ala carte. By ordering ala carte you can easily piece together a meal that meets your nutrition goals. If it is difficult to piece together a reduced calorie meal then plan on taking a doggie bag home, or like some individuals, simply eat half.

If you eat out frequently, look at www.HealthyDiningFinder.com to identify menu items that fit into your eating plan.

A DAY AT A GLANCE

Take time out before you start the day to look at your schedule and the different eating situations you will be confronted with. If you are going to dine out, think about what you will be eating the rest of the day. When you plan your week of menus make sure you include low calorie items to balance the days and meals you may not be able to control. Try not to skip meals; the empty hunger will cause you to eat more. Instead, if you are eating out for dinner, eat a smaller lunch. Plan an afternoon snack to take the edge off your appetite.

FAST FOODS

Fast foods are just that: *fast*. The USDA's research study of 9,000 Americans shows that about a quarter of US adults over the age of 20 eat fast foods and drink twice as many sugary drinks than those who do not. That translates into more calories, fats, carbohydrates, proteins, and added sugars than those that do not. Adding 100 kcal per day can add 10 lbs. to your waistline in one year.

> **High Calories=High Fat:**
> Fat has 9 calories per gram, while carbohydrates and protein only have 4 calories per gram.

Choose smart. The good news is fast foods come in all shapes and sizes and are available just about everywhere. When you're on the road or in a hurry there's nothing wrong with stopping at a fast food restaurant. If you are going to be eating on the road carry a fast food calorie guide. *Calorie King* is a good choice, and can be purchased at most bookstores. (Check the References section of this book for some available guides.) Though fast foods are generally high in calories, fat, and sodium, by using the available nutrition information you can find healthy alternatives. Pay attention to the amount of calories in a serving. The reason most fast foods are high in calories is because they are high in fat. Fat has 9 calories per gram, while carbohydrates and proteins have only 4 calories. So food choices that are high in fat tend to be high calorie items.

An advantage to eating at a fast food restaurant is nutrition information is often available to the consumer. Most fast food restaurants have low calorie healthy items. Subway's menu includes several sandwiches that average 300 calories, so even with a bag of baked chips and a diet soda a lunch can total less than 500 calories. Avoiding the super size items saves calories. A plain hamburger, small fries, and diet coke can also fit into a meal plan. Salads and soups are also available. Piece a meal together by adding up the calories.

MANAGING A MENU

Put together a meal that is enjoyable, healthy, and fits into your calorie budget by using this planning checklist:
1. Try to avoid waiting for a table. Make a reservation and be on time. You can save yourself a few hundred calories by avoiding pre-dinner drinks and appetizers.
2. Think about how you want to "spend" your calories before beginning to scan the menu in a restaurant. You can also research the restaurant's menu ahead of time in order to avoid making an impulsive decision.
3. Review all the menu items available, and work your way through from appetizers to desserts. Choose foods that are healthy and enjoyable. Don't let others pressure you into ordering foods you really don't need or want. Be polite and firm and stick to your plan.
4. Don't be shy about asking how food is prepared. Most restaurants are happy to share this information with you.
5. Modify menu items or substitute low calorie alternatives. Restaurants are used to requests to hold the sauce, go light on the dressing, or put the dressings and gravies on the side. These steps can save you calories.

6. Ask for baked items instead of fried. Most restaurants don't use the "good" fats anyway, so why take in extra fat, especially if it isn't the healthy kind.   There are smart choices you can make about the kind of fat you use.

Remember to determine your hunger level and order your meal accordingly. An appetizer and side dish can be combined to make an entrée.   If the appetizer is small order two appetizers instead of an entire meal. Split your meal with a dining partner, plan to take some home for the next day, or simply leave it. You should be eating until you are satisfied. Listen to your body's signals and become attuned to when you are getting full. Eat slowly and enjoy the company of those you are with.

DRINKS

Regular sodas, lemonade, alcohol, or any beverage that is sweetened can easily add lots of calories. You're better off with a diet beverage or an unsweetened iced tea. You might want to avoid alcohol if it isn't that important to you. Besides, you may find that alcohol stimulates your appetite.

> **Alcohol = 7 calories per gram:**
> **1.5 oz spirits provides approximately**
> **124 calories.**

Since alcohol can make you less aware of what you are eating, you also run the risk of eating more than you had planned. If you do decide to drink, avoid mixed drinks (alcohol mixed with a caloric beverage, such as a soda or fruit juice). A better choice is a glass of red or white wine or hard liquor mixed with a non-caloric beverage such as club soda or diet soda. Ask the bartended to "go easy" on the hard liquor. You can save yourself 100 calories or more a drink.

Learn to limit your alcohol to one drink and sip that drink alternating with water throughout the meal. The calorie level of several drinks can add up quickly and can be equal to the calories of a small meal. Alcohol contains 7 calories per gram. So drinks containing alcohol tend to be high calorie items with little if any nutritional value.

APPETIZERS

Beware of appetizers. They are often high in fat and calories. Many appetizers are fried and breaded making them high calorie items. Sometimes it is best to avoid appetizers entirely.

> **Make a choice:**
> Appetizers or Alcohol, both could up your calories to 200 before starting the meal.

Consider splitting an appetizer with your dining partner. Doing so will save you calories, especially if when choosing an item that isn't loaded with fat and calories. Low calorie items such as soups (broth-based), vegetables, and fruits are good options. Avoid creamy soups, sauces, and dips. Seafood, if it isn't fried, is a good choice. Combining a drink or two and a high calorie appetizer will add as many as 400 calories before you've even started your meal.

LAYER YOUR MEAL

Meal layering is helpful in making you feel fuller with less food. Try to start your meal with a lower calorie, high fiber food. Fresh vegetables, vegetable soup, or a salad with low calorie dressing will fit the bill. The American Journal of Clinical Nutrition reports that people who eat vegetables with a meal actually consume 20 percent fewer calories overall.

> **20-Minute Interval:**
> It takes your brain 20 min. to signal your stomach.

Eat slowly enough to allow for the 20-minute interval where your body signals the brain that there is food in the stomach. If you eat large quantities of food before the 20-minute interval, you are not allowing enough time for your brain to receive the signal that there is food present in the stomach. This leads to overeating.

BREAD

Though the breadbasket seems to be the dieter's demise, who doesn't like a slice of warm crusty French or Italian bread with a meal? Actually a slice of bread contains only 60 to 80 calories and can easily be part of a meal plan. The problem is that limiting yourself to one or two slices often isn't easy. Remember also that adding butter, oil or parmesan cheese can turn an innocent slice of bread into a high calorie item. Try eating a slice of bread without any topping and limiting it to one or two slices.

If your will power takes a beating, ask the waitress to remove the breadbasket or move it away. Providing patrons with a breadbasket is a restaurant's way of keeping you busy while you wait for your meal. Fill the time with water, a low-calorie drink, or conversation. Don't get pressured into eating foods that you really don't want or need. Have a plan and stick to it.

SIDE DISHES

Side dishes are a compliment to an entree and should be modest in portion size. Salads can be foolers. We tend to think of them as low calorie items, and indeed salads without a high calorie dressing can be a good filler before the meal begins. But a low calorie salad can become 250 calories or more if you douse it liberally with dressing.

Most salad dressings are made from fat, particularly the more popular dressings such as ranch, thousand island, and French. A tablespoon of salad dressing contains about 100 calories. Yet who uses just a tablespoon? One tablespoon of Caesar vinaigrette dressing has 70 calories and probably doesn't begin to wet a salad. Choose oil and vinegar dressing or ask to have dressing served on the side so you can control the amount.

Ask about substituting side dishes if the entrée you choose comes with high calorie choices. You can often trade in a double baked potato or fried potatoes for wild rice pilaf, or a plain baked potato, or skip it all together. Choose vegetables without sauces and avoid gravies. Most restaurants will be happy to make the switch for you. Fresh vegetables are low calorie, high in fiber, fill you up, and provide healthy nutrition.

The varieties of entrées to choose from are usually extensive providing an opportunity to eat healthy. Consider the portion size. Pastas are usually served in large quantities. Add a cream sauce and it becomes an even higher calorie item. Ravioli and lasagna meals have fillings and sauces that may make them high in calories. Consider splitting an entrée with a friend or keep half for the next day's lunch. Pasta served with grilled vegetable or with a fresh tomato sauce will save you lots of calories.

A grilled, 16 oz. steak may sound delicious, but it packs a mountain of calories into the one item. The steak alone can provide as many as 800 calories. Instead, try a small 4-6 oz. filet. This can save you as many as 400 calories.

Calories from Steak:
A well marbled steak can be as high as
100 calories per oz.

A half roasted chicken might initially appeal to you as a possible dinner choice. You might think it's a menu item thought of as low calorie and healthy. Yet the reality is this portion is enough for two people, or lunch for two days. If you wouldn't eat half a chicken at home, try to limit the portion size when eating out.

Fresh fish, especially if it's the "special of day" can be a great choice. If you don't like to cook fish at home, ordering it when you eat out provides a healthy and low calorie alternative to many other menu items. Remember, fish contains the right kind of fat. However, be sure you know how it is prepared. Avoid fried fish, especially if coated in a batter. The added calories and fat of batter coated fried fish turns this healthy choice into a calorie nightmare. Grilled and baked fish will save lots of calories. Keep sauces on the side, and eat sparingly. Sauces and toppings are usually made from a fat source and hide the true flavor of foods especially fish. Ask for sauces on the side and use them sparingly.

Design your own meal. Break from tradition and order an appetizer, or a few appetizers to share with friends, to use as your entrée. Try an antipasti plate that comes with a variety of meats, cheese, and olives. A slice of bread, salad, and a glass of wine makes for a great dinner. Tapas are popular and you'll have a fun meal and leave the restaurant not feeling stuffed and guilty about the calories.

DESSERTS

Desserts are an enjoyable ending to a good meal. Again *plan ahead.* Make the decision ahead of time of how to "spend" your calories. Modify your breakfast and lunch that day to accommodate a favorite dessert. When it comes time to ordering dessert think about how hungry you really are, and whether or not you've stuck with your calorie plan for the meal.

Many desserts are high in fat, calories, and sugar plus portions tend to be large. This is a good item to split with someone, or everyone, at the table. If eating at a restaurant known for its decadent chocolate cake and chocolate is your thing, plan to have it. You can save calories from another meal or split a piece of the cake with someone who also loves chocolate but not the calories.

Low calorie choices that are a nice finish to a meal are sorbets, sherbets, and fresh fruit. Some restaurants will offer a frozen yogurt or low-fat ice cream. Sometimes a delicious cup of coffee or tea is a satisfying way to end a meal and is all you really need.

PLANNING IS THE KEY

Busy people, especially those who travel are constantly navigating eating situations. Budgeting daily calories is the most creative way to allow for a variety of foods and to accommodate the many different foods and eating styles you may be challenged with. Planning has also become easier with modern technology and cell phones. There is a new Android and iPhone app (Blackberry app to come soon), called My fitness pal, that has a database of over 726,000 food and restaurant items, including multicultural foods. By planning in advance, you can eat out sensibly and allow yourself healthy food choices guarding against gaining excessive weight.

Answers to Dining Out questions

1. False. With a little planning, you can eat healthy foods when dining out.
2. False.   Knowing the calorie level of fast foods, allows you to include fast foods in your diet.
3. False.
4. True.
5. False.

MENU GUIDELINES FOR RESTAURANTS

Guidelines for various types of eating places are listed below. These tips will provide you with acceptable cooking methods, food items, and suggestions to enhance healthier choices and reduce calories. These guidelines can be used in restaurants or when ordering out.

AMERICAN

Acceptable methods of cooking	
Barbequed	Marinated
Blackened Cajun	Mesquite-grilled
Charbroiled	Stir-fried
Grilled	
Acceptable items	
Barbeque sauce	Mustard
Cocktail sauce	Honey-mustard
Fajitas	Low-calorie or fat-free salad dressing
Jalapenos	Sautéed onions
Lettuce	Peppers
Tomatoes	Mushrooms
Raw onions	Spicy Mexican beef or chicken
Watch for	
Alfredo sauces	Deep
Bacon	Golden, lightly or crispy
Bread crumbs	Guacamole
Butter	Mayonnaise
Cheeses	Sausage
Cream	Served in a crispy tortilla shell

Cream sauces	Sour cream
Fried items-battered	"Special sauces"

Special requests

Could you put the salad dressing, sauce on the side?
How is this item prepared?
Could I have a baked potato, salad, or steamed vegetables instead of the French fries?
Could you leave the French fries off the plate?
Could I have whole-wheat bread in place of the croissant?

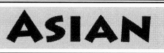

Acceptable methods of cooking

Baked	Simmered
Barbequed	Steamed
Boiled	Stir-fried
Braised	

Acceptable items

Tofu (bean curd)	Fish
Vegetables	Scallops
Shrimp	Chicken
Roast pork	

The below are acceptable for those not watching their sodium intake

✦ Soy	✦ Dipping sauces
✦ Hoisin	✦ Served on a sizzling platter
✦ Brown	✦ Slippery white sauce
✦ Oyster	✦ Velvet sauce
✦ Black bean	✦ Chinese mustard
✦ Hot and spicy tomato	✦ Sweet sauce
✦ Chili	✦ Light wine sauce
✦ Teriyaki sauce	✦ Lobster sauce
✦ Miso	✦ Won ton soup
✦ Hot and Sour soup	

Watch for

Duck	Breaded
Cashews	Crispy
Peanuts	Coconut milk or cream
Water chestnut flour	Foods fried in lard
Chinese noodles	Fried bean curd
Served in a bird's nest	Tempura

Sweet and sour	Agemono
Deep fried	Katsu
Battered	Pan-fried
Special requests	
Could you remove the Chinese noodles from the table?	
Please remove cashews, almonds, or peanuts, or use a small amount.	
Please don't use MSG.	
Could you substitute chicken for the duck?	
Could you omit or reduce the use of oil or soy sauce?	
What type of oil is used in cooking? Could you use peanut oil instead?	

FAST FOODS

Acceptable methods of cooking:	
Baked	
Grilled	
Acceptable items or terms	
Baked potato	Onion
French dip sandwich	Light
Chili	Reduced calorie
Grilled chicken	Fat-free salad dressings
Hamburger (regular, junior, or single)	Low-fat frozen yogurt
Lettuce	Low-fat milk
Tomato	Roast beef
Watch for	
Bacon	Fried chicken
Cheese (any type)	Mayonnaise-based sauces (tartar)
Cheese sauce	Salad dressings
Croissant	Sour cream
Deluxe anything	

Acceptable methods of cooking	
Broiled	Marinated
Demi Glace	Poached
En Papillote	Steamed
Grilled	

Acceptable items	
Au jus	
Bouillabaisse	
Sorbet	
Vinaigrette	

Watch for	
Cheese	Pastry
Au Gratin	Confit
Bechamel	Crème Brulee
Béarnaise	Crème fraiche
Beurre Blanc	Crusted
Buttery	Filet de boef Wellington
Caesar salad	Foie Gras
Canard a l'orange	Gratine
Chateaubriand	Gravy
Coquilles St. Jacques	

Special requests	
Is this item prepared with oil or cream?	
Can it (like butter) be eliminated or reduced?	

GREEK

Acceptable methods of cooking	
Baked	Grilled
Steamed	

Acceptable items	
Soup	Shish-Kabob
Mixed vegetable salads	Tabbouleh
Rice stuffed grape leaves	Plaki

Pita bread without butter or oil	Baba Ghanoush
Roasted eggplant	

Watch for

Pan fried	Nuts
Phyllo dough	Olives
Tahini	Anchovies
Tatziki with full-fat yogurt	Falafel
Hummus	Locanico (sausage)
Goat cheese	Moussaka
Feta	Pastries
Kasseri	

Special requests

May I have pita without oil or butter?	
If oil or butter is added to this dish, can they be omitted or reduced?	

INDIAN

Acceptable method of cooking

Tikka	Cooked or marinated in yogurt
Roasted	Tandoori
Marinated	

Acceptable items

Vegetables	Papadum
Rice	Matta (peas)
Chapti	Indian spices-curry
Naan	Garam
Tomatoes and onions	Marsala
Baked leavened bread	Basmati rice

Watch for

Fried items	Fritters
Pakora	Rayta with full-fat yogurt
Batter dipped	Poori
Somosa	Pappadams
Coconut/coconut milk	Ghee
Cream sauces	Nuts

Special Requests

Please do not garnish with nuts.	
Could I have tea with my meal?	
Could you not salt my meal?	

Acceptable method of cooking	
Marinated	Grilled
Baked	Roasted
Broiled	Sautéed

Acceptable items	
Polenta	Mushroom sauce
Pasta with marinara sauce	Seafood
Pasta with red clam sauce	Tomato-based sauces, marinara
Beans	Bolognese
Medallions	Cacciatore
Vinaigrette	Piccata
Tomatoes	Pasta dishes without cheese
Salads	Fresh clam sauce

Watch for	
Prosciutto	Stuffed shells
Cream sauce	Tortellini
Alfredo sauce	Olives
Four-cheese	Pepperoni
Fried eggplant	Salami
Parmigianino	Pancetta
Pancetta	Manicotti
Carbornara	Lasagna
Francese	Cannelloni
Milanese	Fried Calamari

Special Requests
Could you remove the skin from the chicken?
Could you eliminate the olive oil?
Could I have some tomato sauce for the bread?
Could you hold the Parmesan cheese, bacon, olives, pine nuts, sauce?
Could I have the salad dressing on the side?

LATIN/MEXICAN FOODS

Acceptable methods of cooking	
Sautéed	Blackened
Grilled	Baked
Acceptable items:	
Soft tortillas, corn or flour	Salad
Salsa	Rice
Gazpacho	Burritos without cheese
Vegetable	Ceviche (marinated seafood)
Tortilla	Pinto beans, black beans
Black bean soups	Fish Vera Cruz style
Watch for:	
Fried items	Chiles Rellenos
Enchiladas	Tacos
Guacamole	Flan
Sour cream	Sopaipillas
Refried beans with lard	Nacho
Cheese quesadillas	Chimichangas
Chorizo (Mexican sausage)	
Special requests:	
Could you cut the cheese in half on this item?	
Could you put the guacamole, sour cream, salad dressing on the side?	
Could you take away the chips and salsa?	
Is this dish prepared with oil? Can it be eliminated or reduced?	

UPSCALE RESTAURANTS

Acceptable methods of cooking	
Blackened	Poached
Cajun	Roasted
En brochette (on skewers)	Steamed
Fruit sauce	Tomato
Grilled	Garlic
Marinated	Herb sauces
Mustard sauce, not creamed	
Acceptable items or terms	
Chipotle peppers or sauces	Roasted peppers

Couscous	Salsa-fruit or vegetable
Herbs and spices	Sun-dried tomatoes
Light vinaigrette	Vinegar-balsamic
Polenta	Raspberry
Risotto	
Watch for	
Au gratin	Remoulade sauce
Bacon	Sausage
Butter	Sour cream
Special butters or butter sauces	Stroganoff
Casserole cheese (any)	Whipped cream
Creamed or cream sauces	Wrapped in bacon
Crème fraiche	Pastry shell
Hollandaise sauce	Puffed pastry
Mornay sauce	Phyllo dough
Special requests	
Could you omit or serve the sauce on the side?	
Could you serve the salad dressing on the side?	
Could I have some vinegar or lemon for my salad?	
Could you bring me butter or sour cream for my baked potato on the side?	
Could I have my vegetables steamed rather than sautéed?	

ACCEPTABLE DESSERTS AT ALL RESTAURANTS

Fresh fruit	Sherbet
Sorbet	Angel food cake

ACCEPTABLE SALADS AT ALL RESTAURANTS

Before ordering a salad ask the waiter how the salad is prepared.
Reduce or eliminate bacon, cheese, croutons, olives, and mayonnaise-based items from salads.
Ask for salad dressing on the side.
Vinegar and a light amount of oil or lemon are your best choices for salad dressing.

Remember, when eating out at a restaurant, the portions are generally double what you need. Taking half of the food served home will allow you to enjoy the food twice.

SUPER SIZE: LESS IS BETTER

> **"MODERATION. SMALL HELPINGS. SAMPLE A LITTLE BIT OF EVERYTHING. THESE ARE THE SECRETS OF HAPPINESS AND GOOD HEALTH." - JULIA CHILD**

If you find yourself gaining weight, it might be a good time to review your portion sizes. Often it's not the foods you're eating, but the quantity of food that can get you into trouble and compromise your waistline.

Unfortunately, American portions are becoming a major contributor to weight gain and obesity in this country. Americans are being exposed to a serious case of "Portion Distortion." Many fast-food restaurants offer portions that are from 2 to 8 times greater than portion size from years past. The fast food industry found that by increasing portion sizes, they increase sales and attract new business. "Super size", "Double Gulp", "Hefty Portions", and "Godzilla sizes" describe some of the menu items offered. A study by Pennsylvania State University showed that when portion sizes are increased, individuals tend to eat more. Surprisingly, the study also found that subjects did not feel any fuller after eating a larger portion than with a smaller one.

Restaurants currently serve six ounce bagels, although the standard serving size is two ounces. A Dunkin Donuts bagel is about 330 calories compared to a frozen bagel at the grocery store that averages 160 calories. A typical restaurant size steak is eight ounces, when 3-4 ounces is the standard portion size. When pasta is served in a restaurant, patrons are given approximately three-cup servings, when a half-cup serving is the standard portion size.

McDonald's has increased serving sizes of two of the most popular foods served in America. When McDonalds opened, a small serving of French fries contained 210 calories; while today's super sized order of fries has 540 calories.

When a small cola was originally served it contained 16 ounces and 205 calories. Today, a super sized cola contains 42 ounces and 539 calories. Together these two super sized items comprise 1079 calories, or more than half the daily energy requirement of most Americans.

Even candy bars have grown larger over the years. Years ago, chocolate candy bars contained 0.6 ounces. Today a small bar weighs in at 1.6 ounces and large bars over 6.0 ounces.

Unfortunately if you eat out frequently your perception of what a portion is can become distorted. Some suggestions for determining proper portions include the following:

- ✓ **Purchase convenient measuring cups for liquids and solids, as well as measuring spoons, to determine portion sizes.** Don't use regular cups or spoons that you ordinarily eat from because they are not accurate to measure portions.
- ✓ **Measure out a cup (or a half-cup) of liquid into a glass that you would ordinarily use for your milk or juice.**
    - o Tips:
        1. Use measuring cups for foods such as pasta, rice, soup, or mashed potatoes.
        2. Place the measuring cup on a flat surface and pour the liquid to the line showing the amount you want. If you hold the cup up in the air, the measurement will not be accurate.
        3. Pour the measured amount into an everyday drinking cup and observe the line where the liquid fills. The next time you decide to have a cup of milk, pour the milk into the same glass. Since you know how full a cup should be, this eliminates the need to physically measure the beverage every time.
        4. Allow the same pattern of measuring solid items, such as cereal into a solid measuring cup. After you have measured a cup or half-cup, see where the cereal comes up to on the bowl. Fill the bowl to this point every time you use the item.
- ✓ **Buy a modest kitchen scale to measure solid items that cannot be placed in a cup. This will be helpful to measure meats at home.**

- o Tips:
    1. Meats should be weighed after cooking.
    2. A rule of thumb is that four ounces of raw meat (without a bone) will weigh approximately three ounces cooked.
    3. Five ounces of raw meat with a bone will weigh approximately four ounces cooked.
    4. Estimate the weight of the item before you place it on the scale and then check to see how close you come to the actual portion size

✓ **Getting used to how the foods look on your plate will help you when eating out, rather than carrying scales and measuring cups.**
    - o Tips:
        1. Ask for a doggy bag at the beginning of the meal so that you are not tempted to eat too much.
        2. Since most restaurant portions are greater than what you should normally have, place the leftovers in the doggy bag before beginning the meal.
        3. If you can figure out your portions, you will prevent over-eating.

✓ **Fill your ice cream scoop or soup ladle with water to see how much it holds.**

✓ **Purchase individual bags of an item that remind you of a typical portion size to help you restrict your portions.** When you are done with the bag, you are finished eating the item. Try to eat the item slowly, savoring the taste of the food and enjoying it.

✓ **After several months check your portion sizes again.** This refresher will allow you to make sure that your perception of your portions has not changed. It will also help keep your waistline in check.

VISUALIZING FOOD PORTIONS

To visualize the size of an item or the size of a measuring tool consider the following guidelines:

Portion sizes linked with common household items		
1 Tbs. Peanut Butter or Cream Cheese	=	Three dice or a walnut
1 Ounce of Nuts	=	2 Shot Glasses
1 Ounce of cheese	=	4 Stacked Dice
1 Slice of Cheese	=	3 ½ inch Computer Disk

Portion sizes linked with common household items (Continued)		
1 Chunk of Cheese	=	2 Dominoes Thick
1 Medium Potato	=	Computer Mouse
1 Small Banana	=	Eyeglass Case
1 Medium Apple, Pear, or Peach	=	Tennis Ball
1 Cup Broccoli	=	Light Bulb
1 Cup Cereal	=	Halfway up side of Standard Bowl
½ Chicken Breast, 1 Medium Pork Chop, 1 Small Hamburger, 1 Fish Fillet	=	Deck of Cards
1 Small Chicken Leg or Thigh	=	2 Ounces
½ Cup Tuna, Cottage Cheese or Pasta	=	Hockey Puck
½ Cup Grapes	=	Light Bulb

Food portions can also be visualized using your hand as a measurement guide		
One fruit serving	=	Finger length diameter
1 tsp. butter, margarine, or peanut butter size	=	Top half of your thumb
One cup of pasta, cereal, cooked vegetables	=	Fist volume
Serving of nuts	=	One Handful
Small potato	=	Half of a fist
½ cup fruit, vegetables	=	Palm of hand
One serving of snack foods	=	Two Handfuls
One 4-ounce portion of meat, fish, Poultry	=	Palm of hand
One ounce or one tablespoon	=	Thumb volume
One teaspoon	=	Thumb tip

Portion Control Plates, Bowls, & Food Scales	
Potion Control Dinnerware	http://www.preciseportions.com
	http://www.diabetesandmore.com
Portion Control Bowls & Plates	Measure Up Bowl Set, "Measup 2" at Target or 800-678-5752
	Slimware Plate set with 4 plates at 800-678-5752
Kitchen Scales, food scales, and cooking scales	http://www.oldwillknottscales.com

Rate Your Plate with the Food Groups

It's tough to decide how much food to put on your plate. Let this be your guide! Servings should fit within a 9" plate, or the inner center of a large dinner plate. Go to www.ChooseMyPlate.com to determine your individual calories and servings. The basic daily requirements to keep in mind are:

Food Group	Daily Requirement	One Serving Size Equal to
Grains	5 ounces, ½ should be whole grains	1 slice of bread 1 cup of cereal ½ cup cooked rice, cooked pasta or cooked cereal
Vegetables	2 cups	1 cup raw or cooked vegetables or vegetable juice 2 cups raw leafy greens counts as 1 cup
Fruit	1 ½ cups	½ cup dried fruit 1 cup of fruit 1 small apple (4 oz.) 1 small banana (4 oz.)
Milk	3 cups	1 ½ ounces of natural cheese 2 ounces processed cheese ¾ cup of plain non-fat yogurt
Meat and Beans	5 ounces	1 ounce of meat, poultry or fish ¼ cup cooked dry beans 1 egg 1 tablespoon of peanut butter ½ ounce nuts or seeds
Oils	5 teaspoons	1 teaspoon oil: Canola, Olive, Peanut 10 Peanuts 2 teaspoons peanut butter Mixed nuts, 6 nuts equal 1 teaspoon Olives: 8 large black olives or 10 large green olives 1/8th of an avocado

RATE YOUR PLATE USING THE PLATE METHOD

Carbohydrates

Carbohydrates include starchy vegetables (like potatoes) and grains (like whole wheat bread and rice or whole wheat pasta). Carbohydrates at breakfast are greater than for lunch and dinner. Using MyPlate guidelines, choose two servings per meal from grains or starchy vegetables that fit nicely into ¼ of a 9 inch plate for lunch and dinner.

Vegetables

Fill half your plate with non-starchy vegetables, like broccoli, cauliflower, green beans, or carrots. Also, green leafy vegetables, such as salad, counts as a serving of vegetables.

Protein

Keep meat choices to 3-4 ounces twice daily. Meat and Bean choices, shown on the MyPlate guidelines, give ideas for serving sizes for the different types of protein.

Dairy

One cup of milk per meal, or an equivalent, will do it! This requirement ensures there is sufficient calcium in your diet. Dairy also provides protein and carbohydrate.

Fruit

You might find it difficult to eat this much food. If so, save your fruit serving for snacks. Fruit is portable and easy to put in a backpack or briefcase.

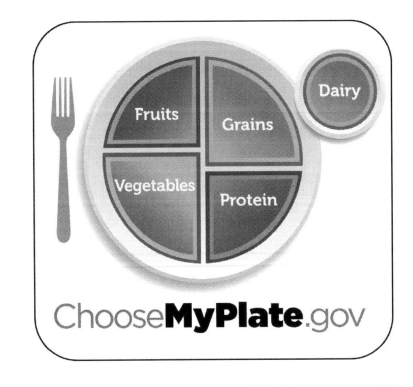

VACATIONS

For most of us, vacations are viewed as a 'time out' from the busyness of our daily routines. A time to kick back, relax, and indulge. But who wants a great time ruined by returning with the extra pounds you may have fought to lose? Think positive. Vacations are a reprieve from our fast paced life. A little planning and you can avoid packing on the pounds. You might even lose a few pounds.

We decided to do a little soul searching. Our motto: same rules apply everywhere; all the time. In other words we stick to a meal schedule and continue exercising. In fact, if we think we'll be eating more, we increase our activity. Seeing a city on foot is a great way to build in exercise. We surveyed individuals who don't gain when on vacation and here's what they said:

1. Many individuals look for vacations with built in exercise, walking, hiking, biking, and swimming/snorkeling.
2. Some said they avoid hotels and instead rent a condo, house, or apartment. They can shop and prepare some meals, saving time, money, and calories.
3. On road trips or long flights individuals pack snacks, energy bars, sandwiches.
4. For those staying in hotels, they make sure a refrigerator is available and head to the nearest grocery store for healthy foods/snacks.
5. If it isn't an outdoor vacation, individuals make sure they stay where exercise equipment is available.

6. Individuals staying with relatives try to help plan and shop for meals. This allows them to stay on their diet plan and help out their hosts with the extra costs of having guests.
7. Cruises can become food orgies. Sticking to a meal schedule and avoiding impulse eating is critical. Most increase activity on board ship, signing up for exercise classes, swimming, or walking the ship.
8. Many say they have a drink quota, knowing that calories in a few pina coladas or margaritas add up quickly.
9. When individuals eat all their meals at restaurants, they look for low calorie menus, avoiding fried and breaded foods and opting for fresh simply prepared meals.
10. Many individuals simply split their meals or desserts with their traveling companion.

Check your weight before leaving on a vacation and when returning. If there is a scale available, check your weight half way through the vacation. Scales keep you focused and honest.

OFFICE FOOD

Office food seems to be here, there and anywhere and can sabotage healthy eating efforts. Whether it be trying to lose weight or attempting to eat more healthfully, office food does no one any favors.

Office food usually consists of the ever present candy jar on the desk of your boss, the receptionist, or other well-meaning food providers. It is also the breakfast donuts, cookies, birthday cakes, holiday leftovers, and school fundraiser candy and cookies.

A recent study reported in The International Journal of Obesity showed that individuals at work ate an average of 5.6 pieces of fun-sized candy if placed in a see-through container. If the container was opaque, this was reduced to 3.1 pieces daily. If an individual is sitting close to the candy dish, they add an average of 2.1 pieces daily. Adding only 2 pieces daily of fun-sized candy, without any exercise or dietary change amounts to an increase of 7 pounds each year. Having the candy jar around the office is also quite costly amounting to an annual cost of $546.

HOW TO AVOID THE CALORIE TEMPTERS AND WEIGHT DESTROYERS

- Bring in healthy snacks that are planned into your diet plan to reduce your urge to splurge.

- Talk to your Human Relations manager about including weight and exercise programs in your company benefits. Encourage them to suggest removal of candy jars and removal of unhealthy food in common areas. Have employees compete for weight loss and exercise program prizes to encourage adherence to programs.

- When sales representatives ask what items they can bring to the office, suggest fruit and other healthy snacks. If they bring in lunch, ask if you can suggest healthy items they can bring or healthy eating places that they can find healthy choices.

- Drink a hot low calorie beverage to reduce your desire for a high calorie treat. These would include: coffee, tea, low calorie cocoa, or low calorie apple cider.

- Drink a cold low calorie beverage such as: iced tea, ice water, seltzer water, or diet pop to cut down your consumption of high calorie snacks. Stopping to drink either a cold or hot beverage gives you a chance to stop and think through a high calorie choice.

- Ask the candy stasher to put the candy in a drawer.

- Reduce office birthday parties to once monthly and suggest a healthy luncheon to your boss in place of the high calorie birthday cake.

- Remind bosses that stopping by the candy jar increases time fraternizing, decreases time spent on work, increases the chance of employee health risks and obesity, and increases health insurance costs.

HOLIDAY EATING, FOOD & FUN

Holidays are a celebration of family, friends, and food. If you've stopped to read this chapter, you may be one that dreads the challenges that accompany holiday eating. For some, extra holiday eating begins around Halloween. For others, it's Thanksgiving that marks the beginning of holiday overeating. We hear it all the time, "I haven't stopped eating since I bought candy for the trick or treaters."

> Remember: Eat, Drink and be WARY!!

Let's face it! The holidays can be stressful, and for some emotionally difficult. Life tends to be busy enough and then suddenly the holidays arrive. Busy days become even busier and our routine takes a backseat to all the demands. Indulging in favorite foods this time of year couldn't be easier or more tempting. Though the next 6 to 8 weeks are tough for most of us, we're confident that if you follow some simple rules, do a little calorie budget planning, and have a "no weight gain" motto you'll enter January the same weight as you were before the holidays began.

For starters, be prepared for the party by identifying low calorie snacks to choose and the foods to limit or avoid by bringing along your favorite low calorie foods to enjoy and share with others.

"What's on the Menu?"

Holiday Snacks to Choose
•   Raw veggies, limiting dips to 2 tablespoons
•   Most hard candies
•   2 Alcoholic Beverages for Men, 1 Alcoholic Beverage for Women
Wine: one serving is equal to 5 oz.
Beer: one serving is equal to 12 oz.
Spirits: one serving is equal to 1 1/2 oz.
•   Mixers for Spritzers: Sugar Free carbonated beverages, Water, Seltzer Water

Snacks to Eat in Moderation
Appetizers: don't pile them on the plate; limit the assortment to one small appetizer plate.
Salad dressing and dips, limit to 2 tablespoons
Fruits, limit to 1/4 cup
Junk food: limit Chips, Cheese Curls, Corn Chips, etc. to 1/4 cup
Cookies: choose 1 or 2 small cookies, no more

Avoid these Goodies!
Chocolate, anything: Cakes, small cookies, fudge are loaded with calories
Appetizers with Cheese/Meats, including cheese spreads
Nuts, it's too easy to overindulge
Junk food: Crackers, Potato Chips, Cheese Curls, Corn Chips, etc.
Egg Nog, especially with alcohol
Mixers: Juices, Regular Soda

These are tips we use, and provide our clients, to help maintain weight through the holiday season.   Choose a few or all of them.   Write them down on a day planner or "to do" list as a consistent reminder of your goals.

Helpful Tips to Maintaining Weight through the Holiday Season
1. <u>Check your weight frequently</u>. Forget about losing weight during the holidays. Instead, commit to maintaining your weight. By weighing several times a week during the toughest weeks, you'll be able to quickly identify any weight gain and develop a strategy to lose or curb those pounds from adding up.
2. <u>Stay active</u>. That's right, don't stop exercising. In fact, if you are eating more calories you'll need to increase your activity/exercise. Try climbing stairs at work or walking during your lunch hour.
3. <u>Favorite Foods</u>. Plan to have some of your favorite foods. Deprivation backfires and leads to overeating when your guard is down.
4. <u>Snack Healthy before the Party</u>. Never go to a party or out to dinner hungry. Eat a high fiber or high protein snack 1-2 hours before the party. These snacks will take the edge off your appetite and make it easier to stick to your plan.
5. <u>Budget Calories for Alcohol</u>. Decide ahead of time how much alcohol you will drink. Have a budget of calories to spend on alcohol. Avoid eggnogs and mixed holiday drinks. Instead drink lite beer, champagne, or wine spritzer. Switch to a diet beverage after you've spent your alcohol calories.
6. <u>Eat the Foods you Enjoy</u>. Eat the foods you enjoy on the main holiday and skip them during the rest of the season. Extra pounds come from days of overeating, not from overeating at a single meal or on a single day. Maintain or adjust your usual eating pattern as much as you can on the other days.
7. <u>Keep Low-Calorie Snacks on Hand</u>. Make sure you keep low calorie alternatives at home, the workplace, and at parties. Between meal snacking is a challenge during the holidays because of increased availability of high-calorie foods. Always have low calorie choices available to munch on that will keep you away from the infinite parade of cookies and candies.
8. <u>Keep a Calorie Budget</u>. Make all your meals meet your calorie budget and save some extra calories for social eating. Every pound on the scale is equal to 3500 extra calories.
9. Fill an appetizer plate with foods you like and <u>move away from the buffet table</u>.
10. <u>Use an Appetizer Size Plate</u>. If you fill a smaller plate with the foods you enjoy, and don't go back for seconds, you'll eat less.
11. <u>Follow the Vacation Eating Guidelines</u>. If you're staying with family and friends make sure you have foods on hand that fit into your eating style. Bring foods along or take time out to shop when you arrive.
12. <u>Plan a Time-Out</u>. Most people complain they overeat when they're tired. Try a short nap, yoga, or a few minutes of quiet time.
13. <u>Hang out with a normal weight individual at a party</u>. Chances are you'll eat less.

Remember, holidays are about family, friends, and fun. Keeping track of calories, staying within a personal calorie budget, and watching your weight will allow you to maintain your weight and still enjoy the foods of the holiday without the guilt.

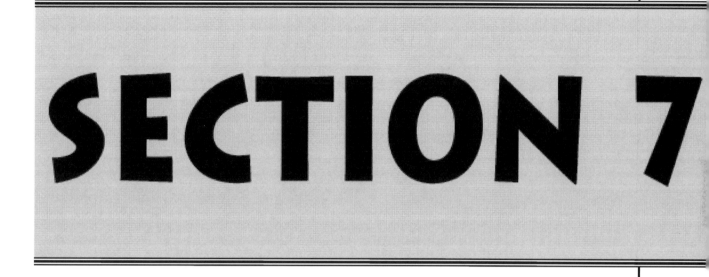

SECTION 7

DEALING WITH POPULAR FOODS SENSIBLY

BEVERAGES

Sugar-sweetened beverage consumption has doubled in the last twenty years contributing to obesity in this country. It has been estimated that twenty percent of the calories consumed in the American diet are from beverages. A major problem is that beverages do not provide the same sense of fullness that food does. This lack of satiety with beverages can result in high caloric consumption especially when combined with high calorie foods. Another area of concern is that the beverage glasses being served are often extremely oversized. At fast food restaurants it is not uncommon to be offered a quart of a high-calorie beverage. This amount can add approximately 480 calories to your daily intake.

Recent beverage recommendations were made by a panel of nutritionists in the March 8, 2006 issue of American Journal of Clinical Nutrition. Concern has arisen about new beverage consumption because federal guidelines and the new MyPlate focus on food and not on beverages.

The nutritionists recommended the following daily limits for adults

- Unsweetened tea or coffee- up to 40 ounces
- Sugar-sweetened soda, juice, or drinks- no more than 8 ounces
- Low-fat or skim milk and soy beverages- up to 16 ounces
- Diet soda and other non-caloric drinks- up to 32 ounces
- Alcoholic beverages, one drink for women daily and two drinks for men daily:
  - A drink equals 12 ounces beer
  - 5 ounces wine
  - 1.5 ounces spirits

Americans are encouraged to drink primarily water and limit calorie containing beverages. Unsweetened tea and coffee are considered acceptable substitutes for water. Beverage consumption should be limited to 10 percent to 14 percent of daily calories, which is half the amount presently consumed in this country. Common beverages, frozen drinks, and Starbucks drinks are included for review.

It is apparent that these frequently consumed products are significantly contributing to the increased caloric intake by Americans. Be careful when consuming these beverages. Try to pick non-caloric beverages that will add zero calories to your daily intake. Although beverages can go down very quickly and do not seem to have many calories, remember that their caloric contribution is significant. Watching your caloric fluid intake can make the difference in maintaining your ideal body weight or if you are struggling to lose weight.

Caloric contents of beverages (serving size = 8oz.)	
Whole Milk	170 calories
2% Milk	125 calorie
Skim Milk	90 calories
Lemonade	99 calories
Punch	96 calories
Snapple	100 calories
Diet Snapple	20 calories
Orange juice	120 calories

DIGESTING THE BAR FACTS

Energy bars are convenient, small, with little clean up required. The problem is the huge selection offered. So which do you choose? This depends solely on your preferences and needs. Some are looking for a snack, others use energy bars to replenish fuel after a long period of exercise. Some use energy bars as a meal replacement, and others simply like the taste and convenience. Remember "Energy" also means calories. Energy bars are another way to consume calories in a quick neat little package. Energy bars themselves will not provide magical powers to boost brain power nor will they turn anyone into an Olympic athlete. The bottom line... they provide calories.

Whatever your reason for choosing an energy bar it is important to consider these factors...

- Check the label calories, these bars can range from 100- 400 calories.

- Choose a bar that is low in fat; less than 5 g is reasonable.

- To replenish fuel during or after exercise look for bars with at least 25 g of carbohydrates.

- When strength training and working muscles, look for bars with at least 25g of protein.

- Meal replacement bars should contain proportionately higher amounts of carbohydrates, protein, and fiber.

- Look at the sugar content; these can contain just as much sugar as a candy bar. Remember 1 tsp. of sugar is equal to 4 grams of sugar.

- If you consume multiple bars a day you may be getting more vitamins and minerals than you need.

- Have some real food as a snack for variety; fruit is a great choice.

- Energy bars cannot be counted on to provide your daily fiber need. Isolated fibers, such as inulin, chicory, and oligosaccharides, may not provide the same benefit as fiber offered from food.

HOW DOES YOUR ENERGY BAR STACK UP?

Name	Type of bar ✖	Calories ⚙	Fat ⚙	Sat. fat ⚙	Fiber ⚙	Pro ⚙	Carbs ⚙
Advantage Bar	NB,HP, LC	230	10	3	2	20	3
Balance	NB	200	6	3.5	<1	14	22
Bear Valley Meal Pack	MR, HC	400	12	2	6	16	56
Biochem Ultimate low-carb	NB, HC	240	7	1	0	23	2
Biochem Ultimate protein	MR, HP	290	5	4	0	30	19
Biox	MR, HP, HC	330	3	2	3	27	48
Body Smarts Bar	NB, HC	200	5	4.5	2	5	33
Boost Bar	S, HC	190	6	3.5	2	4	29
Boulder Bar	NB, HC	210	4	1	3	8	37
Bumble Bar	NB	230	16	2	5	6	17
Carb Options	NB	200	8	4	.5	16	17
Cliff Bar 🌿	NB, HC	240	4	1	5	10	41
EAS Results for women	S, HC, W	190	6	2	4	11	28
Energx cookies	NB, HC	200	3	1	4	15	31

Name	Type of bar ✖	Calories	Fat ○	Sat. fat ○	Fiber ○	Pro ○	Carbs ○
Fiber One	S,HC	150	4.5	2	9	3	28
Figurines	MR, HC	280	11	3	2	12	34
Gatorade Bar	MR, HC	260	5	1	1	7	47
Genisoy	NB, HC	230	4.5	3	2	14	33
Glucerna Bar	S	150	4	3	1	6	25
Glucerna Mini Bar	S	80	2.5	1	< 1	4	12
Honey Stinger Bar	S	180	5	2	2	10	27
Jenny Craig	NB, HC	220	5	4	1	10	33
Kashi Go Lean	MR, HC	280	5	3	7	14	47
Larabar Apple Pie	S (gluten-free, vegan, & kosher)	190	10	1	5	4	24
Lean Body	MR, HP	300	7	6	0	30	19
Luna	S, HC	180	4	3	2	10	26
Met-RX cereal bar	MR, HC	290	3	1	4	25	43
Met-RX ⚡	MR, HP, HC	320	2.5	0.5	0	27	48
Met-RX energy ⚡	MR, HP, HC	340	4	2	0	27	50
Met-RX protein plus	MR, HP, HC	290	4	3	3	32	31
Mojo	NB	200	7	.05	2	9	25
Myoplex	MR, HP, HC	340	7	2	2	24	44
Natural Vitality's New You	S, HC, W	170	3	1.5	3	10	26
Odwalla bar	NB, HC	240	5	1	3	16	31
Odwalla super protein	MR, HC	260	7	2	4	9	44
Parillo bar	NB, HC	230	6	0	3	14	35
Peak bar	MR, HC	314	6	1	3	5	58
Power Bar original ⚡	NB, HC	230	2	0.5	3	10	45
Power Bar Protein Plus ⚡	MR, HP, HC	290	5	2.5	1	24	38
PR Bar	NB	200	6	2	0	13	23
Pria	S, W	110	3	2.5	<1	5	17
Promax	MR, HC	290	6	3.5	1	20	38
Protein 21	MR, HP, HC	290	5	3.5	2	21	40
Pure Protein	MR, HP, HC	260	4.5	3.5	1	31	27

Name	Type of bar ✖	Calories	Fat ⚙	Sat. fat ⚙	Fiber ⚙	Pro ⚙	Carbs ⚙
Sci-Fit	MR, HP	334	5	4	1	35	22
Slim Fast ⭔	S	140	5	2	2	5	20
Soy Joy Bar	S	130	5	2.5	3	4	17
Trek Bar	S, HC	130	2	0	3	3	29
Twinlab Ironman	NB	230	8	2	0	16	23
Twinlab Protein	MR, HP	340	5	4	0	35	12
Twinlab Soy	S	180	6	3	5	15	22
Twinlab Ultrafuel	NB, HC	230	0	0	2	15	42
Ultra Slim-fast breakfast	S, HC	170	0	0	2	1	39
Ultra Slim-fast snack ⭔	S	120	4	0	3	2	19
Weight Watchers Snack	S	120	4	2	3	2	23
You Are What You Eat	S, HC	190	3.0	1.0	5	4	42
Zone Perfect	NB	210	7	3.5	2	14	24

⚙ - Grams (g) of nutrient

⭔ -Nutrition content dependent on variety and flavor

✖ -

S	Snack	Up to 199 calories
NB	Nutrition Bar	200-250 calories
MR	Meal Replacement	>250 calories
HC	High Carbohydrate	>25g
HP	High Protein	>20g
LC	Low Carbohydrate	<5g
W	Made for Women	Women's formula

PIZZA

Pizza is a popular American food that is currently a $30 billion a year industry. Pizza can be a healthy addition to your diet if you make sensible selections. If not, two slices of pizza can add over 800 calories and a day's worth of sodium, cholesterol, and saturated fat to your intake. The popularity of pizza can add to the high incidence of heart disease in this country and our bulging waistlines.

A typical unhealthy pizza choice is Domino's Hand Tossed Pepperoni Pizza. One slice is equivalent to a McDonald's Egg McMuffin. Pizza Hut's Stuffed Crust Meat Lover's Pizza is equal to a McDonald's Big Mac, and who eats just one slice?

Frozen pizza plays a big part in the typical American's diet. It is currently the number one frozen dinner choice in this country. With the focus on improving food choices to reduce the incidence of obesity, many companies are beginning to offer more healthful pizza choices. Look at pg. 244 for some of these better choices for frozen pizza.

There are a number of healthy reasons to include pizza in your diet. Pizza sauce is rich in lycopene, an antioxidant that protects individuals against prostrate and cervical cancers and reduces heart disease. It is also helps prevent eye disorders such as macular degeneration and cataracts that can lead to blindness. Pizza is a good source of lycopene due to its tomato sauce base. Cooked tomatoes contain 10 mg lycopene which is more than fresh tomatoes. Vegetable pizzas, such as spinach, broccoli, and pepper can supply health benefits with their added contents of beta-carotene, folate, vitamin C, calcium, vitamin K, and anti-oxidants.

Cheese is a high source of calcium helpful in maintaining healthy teeth and bones. One slice of pizza can supply approximately 20% of the daily need for calcium. To reduce the fat and cholesterol content of pizza, look for part-skim mozzarella which is leaner than traditional pizza cheeses. Many strict vegetarians choose soy cheese on their pizzas. Soy cheese has no cholesterol, lower saturated fat, and lower calories per slice. It is also helpful in lowering cholesterol levels in the body.

Pizza crust can be made with trans fats that increase heart disease risk. To insure a healthy crust, look for those made with whole wheat, oat bran, and wheat germ. Stay away from crusts with shortening and partially hydrogenated vegetable oil.

Pizza can also supply over 30 percent of your recommended daily allowance for sodium in one slice. Excessive sodium intake can be a concern because it has been linked with high blood pressure and increased risk of stomach cancer. The adult recommended daily limit for sodium is 2400 mg. Compare pizza brands to ensure that a serving does not contain over 800 mg sodium. Make sure on days you choose pizza you limit your use of convenience foods, fast foods, and prepared foods that supply high amounts of sodium.

Suggestions for improving your pizza choices include:
- Order your pizza with half the cheese. Choose vegetable toppings that are lower in calories and higher in nutrition. Some companies add extra cheese with vegetable pizzas so make sure to check the calories. Chicken and ham are the next best choices. Try to avoid high-fat choices such as sausage, pork, and beef. Pepperoni is a better choice than these if the rest of your group is pushing meat pizzas. Another option would be to order half the pizza with meat and half without. This allows calorie and fat hungry friends their choice and you get yours. If meat pizza is a favorite, having one slice with and one slice without will lower your calories, fat, and cholesterol intake.
- Avoid "Stuffed Pizza" where cheese is injected into the pizza's crust. This unnecessary addition will boost calories, cholesterol, and saturated fat.
- Order a salad with low calorie dressing with your pizza. This will fill you up and will allow you to stick to one piece of pizza instead of two or three.
- Avoid other side orders that are often offered at pizzerias. These include: Buffalo wings, bread sticks, and garlic bread.

Brand	Calories/ Serving	Fat/Saturated Fat/Cholesterol	Carbs, Protein, Sodium
A.C. LaRocco Tomato &Feta	251	7gm Fat 2 gm Saturated Fat 11 mg Cholesterol	39 grams Carbohydrate 11 grams Protein 341 mg Sodium
Amy's Pizza Cheese	305	12 grams Fat 4 grams Saturated Fat 15 mg Cholesterol	39 grams Carbohydrate 12 grams Protein 600 mg Sodium
Tombstone Original Pizza, Extra Cheese	293	13 grams Fat 6 grams Saturated Fat 30 mg Cholesterol	32 grams Carbohydrate 14 grams Protein 586 mg Sodium
DiGiorno Rising Crust Spinach, Mushroom, & Garlic Pizza	262	8grams Fat 3 grams Saturated Fat 17 mg Cholesterol	35 grams Carbohydrate 12 grams Protein 664 mg Sodium
Freshetta DiGiorno Brick Oven Fire Baked Crust Roasted Portobello Mushrooms & Spinach	273	9 grams Fat 4 grams Saturated Fat 19 mg Cholesterol	36 grams Carbohydrate 11 grams Protein 602 mg Sodium
Wolfgang Puck Wood-Fired Thin Crust Vegetable	221	7 grams Fat 3 grams Saturated Fat 20 mg Cholesterol	29 grams Carbohydrate 12 grams Protein 449 mg Sodium
California Pizza Kitchen Barbequed Chicken	287	9 grams Fat 5 grams Saturated Fat 31 mg Cholesterol	34 grams Carbohydrate 17 grams Protein 717 mg Sodium
Freshetta Southwest Style Chicken Supreme with Roasted Red Peppers	302	10 grams Fat 4 grams Saturated Fat 21 mf Cholesterol	40 grams Carbohydrate 13 grams Protein 965 mg Fat
Red Baron Pizzeria Style Special Deluxe	319	14 mg Fat 5 grams Saturated Fat 20 mg Cholesterol	36 grams Carbohydrate 14 grams Protein 824 mg Sodium

SAUSAGE	Dominos 12 inch	Dominos 14 inch	Pappa John's 14 inch	Pizza Hut 12 inch
Portion	1/8 pizza	1/8 pizza	1/8 pizza	1/8 pizza
Carbohydrate (grams)	30	24	24	
Protein (grams)	7	12	13	16
Fat (grams)	10	13	18	18
Calories	191	267	303	340
Cholesterol (mg)	28.5	28.5	31	30
Sodium (mg)	558	587	724	910

VEGETABLE	Dominos 12 inch	Dominos 14 inch	Pappa John's 14 inch	Pizza Hut 12 inch
Portion	1/8 pizza	1/8 pizza	1/8 pizza	1/8 pizza
Carbohydrate (grams)	28	39	24	29
Protein (grams)	9.5	13.2	9	9
Fat (grams)	8	11	11	8
Calories	220	302	228	220
Cholesterol	17	38	14	5
Sodium	49	684	447	580

SUSHI

Sushi is a popular Japanese food that has become very popular in the United States. It can be found in grocery stores, restaurants, and bars. It is also a food that can be eaten on the run. Sushi can be cold, cooked, or topped with sweet vinegar. It is often filled with raw, cooked, or marinated fish. Shellfish, eggs, or vegetables can also be used for fillers.

Sushi can be made in a variety of ways including hand-formed, rolled, or pressed. It can be made into small bite-sized pieces or large rolls. It is often made with sliced raw fish called sashimi.

Sushi is a nutritious food that is low in calories, low in sodium when limited condiments are used, and low fat unless fried or very fatty fish are used. It is an excellent source of carbohydrate, protein, and other nutrients depending on the types used. Check the lists below for your best choices and those items you should look out for.

Good Choices:

- Try sushi served steamed, grilled, or boiled.
- Use low sodium soy sauce or Tamari sauce or limit use of added condiments to minimize sodium intake.
- Choose reputable restaurants, grocery stores, or bars to insure that the raw fish you are eating is fresh. A few tips for ensuring the safety of fish is to go to places that have a large customer base. This will increase the chances that the fish served or sold is being turned over fast. Take a look in the kitchen on the way to the restroom. Does it look clean and

neat? Fresh sushi should have a clean water smell. If the fish you are being served has a fishy smell, it is probably not fresh and should be avoided. Does the restaurant or fish store have a fishy smell? This also probably means that the fish is not fresh.

- Order steamed veggies like hijiki (cooked sea weed) or Ooshitashi (boiled spinach) with soy sauce to fill up.
- Pick soups and sashimi that tend to be lower in calories.
- Choose sushi that is made with shrimp, eel, or crab, scrambled eggs, tofu, or vegetables.
- Consider sukiyaki that is meat or vegetables usually served at the table in a shallow pan or
- Teppanyaki dishes that are meat, fish, or vegetables cooked on an iron griddle.
- Order brown rice in place of white rice because it retains many nutrients that are lost in processing white rice. These include: iron, vitamin B, vitamin B3, and Magnesium. Brown rice wrapped in nori (dried seaweed) has iodine, zinc, cilium, vitamins A, E, C, and K. It is also higher in fiber and protein.
- Wasabi sauce (hot green paste) is a Japanese horse radish that is served with sashimi. It can help you from having food poisoning due to its antimicrobial properties.
- Ginger is served with sushi in a pickled form to cleanse the palate after each sushi piece. Ginger contains the compounds gingerols and shogaols that stimulate digestive juices and neutralize stomach acids. Ginger is effective in blocking the body's vomit reflex. It also helps lower cholesterol and limits blood clotting like aspirin.
- Mackerel is a great sushi choice due to its omega-3 fatty acids, low mercury levels, and selenium levels that work along with the omegas to neutralize free radicals.
- Drink green tea as your beverage to help lower total cholesterol and improve the ratio of HDL (good cholesterol) to LDL (bad cholesterol). It is also a zero calorie choice.

WATCH OUT FOR
- Be careful with tempura vegetables or seafood that are cooked in batter and deep-fried. This choice can add extra calories, fat, and cholesterol depending on the type of oil used.
- Stay clear of teriyaki or yaketori sauce that both have a considerable amount of sugar that can add calories.
- Sake can add a considerable amount of calories having 40 calories/ ounce.

- Avoid spicy items that tend to be higher in calories and fat due to the sauces that usually have added mayonnaise.
- Restrict use of red bluefish tuna due to its high mercury content and (PCB's), organic compounds that can cause harm to the brain and endocrine system.
- Avoid tobiko sushi that is made of fish roe and quail eggs due to the high cholesterol and saturated fat content. Since they are eaten raw, there is a risk of salmonella poisoning.

The FDA has recommended that individuals who are pregnant or those with compromised immune systems should avoid the use of raw fish. These would include children, elderly, and those with liver disease, diabetes, and other autoimmune disorders. This is due to the higher risk of severe outcomes from infection from spoiled raw fish.

	Serving Size	Calories	Carbohydrate (grams)	Protein (grams)	Fat (grams)	Sodium (grams)
California roll	4 pieces	150	25	4	4	170
Dragon roll	4 pieces	290	28	10	3	300
Shrimp nigri	4 pieces	130	18	12	1	620
Shrimp tempura roll	6 pieces	220	12	10	13	500
Cooked soybeans	½ cup	100	9	8	3	310
Spicy salmon roll	6 pieces	160	16	8	7	560
Spicy tuna roll	6 pieces	100	16	8	7	430
Spider roll (soft-shelled crab)	3 pieces	200	20	11	9	620
Summer roll	1 roll	130	14	10	9	90
Vegetable roll	5 pieces	120	22	3	3	520

MOVIE, FAIR, AND CARNIVAL FARE

Buttered popcorn is by far the most popular snack choice at movie theaters. Each weekend millions of people worldwide consume large amounts of popcorn at movie theaters. Movie popcorn is a potential problem food, due to its large portion size and fake "butter". This "butter" is a combo of hydrogenated coconut and soy bean oil with beta-carotene added for color. This concoction is high in cholesterol, salt, fat, and trans fat. Making healthier movie theater snack choices can be a rewarding task.

Portion control is the essential key to successful weight management. A small bag of movie popcorn holds about 7 cups and approximately 500 calories. A large tub of movie theater popcorn can total a whopping 1,500 calories, not to mention any other beverages or snacks added. A large popcorn without movie "butter" has the potential to contain about 80 grams of fat, with more than 50 grams saturated fat. On the other hand, if you succumb to the "butter" the fat escalates up to 130 grams, which equates to around four McDonald Big Macs.

Watching your fat intake is a real challenge at the theater. Opting for a smaller size, unbuttered popcorn and sharing it with a friend is a great option. Avoid special family combo packages unless you are actually sharing them with a family. Eliminating snack consumption at the movie theater and eating a well balanced meal before arriving can lead to a less tempting theater experience.

Baked bread pretzels with cheese sauce are another popular movie theater snack. A great, and tasty, alternative is to eliminate the cheese sauce and replace it with spicy brown mustard.

Instead of snacking on candy, bring a small bag of finger fruits like strawberries, grapes, or berries. Healthy dry cereal can be a great option, and can keep you munching at much lower calories.

CARNIVAL, FAIR, & STADIUM FOODS

Carnival, fair, and ball game food can be particularly high in calories and poor in nutrition. Check out the calories and nutrition information listed. If you look forward to a particular food at a favorite event try the following:
1. Eat smaller meals leading up to the snack.
2. Use some of your snack calories to put towards the treat.
3. Share the snack with another person.

Know what you're getting into before you go! Have fun and still keep to your calorie goals.

Food	Carbohydrate (grams)	Protein (grams)	Fat (grams)	Calories (kcal)
1/3 lb. hot dog	31	14	41	550
Foot long hot dog	41	18	26	470
Corndog (4 oz)	36	8	21	250
French fries (7 oz.)	70	16	24	560
Cheese fries (10 oz.)	62	14	38	645
Onion Rings (3)	40	8	13	310
Cole Slaw (5 oz.)	37	3	21	350
Kettle Corn (5 oz.)	110	6	15	600
Kettle Corn (10 oz.)	220	12	30	1200
Funnel Cake, Plain	80	11	44	760
Funnel Cake, Cinnamon/sugar	88.5	11	44	790
Strawberries and Cream	96		8	830
Churro (1 oz)	21	9	8	165
Cotton Candy (5 ½ oz.)	156			625
Soft Pretzel (4 ½ oz.)	70	10.5	2	240
Soft Pretzel (8 oz.)	147	20.7	5	710
Candied Apple (7 oz.)	80		0.5	330
Snow Cone (3 oz.)	68			270
Slushie (16oz.)	65			260
Malt (16 oz.)	85		33	690

It is better to think of creative and lower calorie ways to enjoy your favorite snacks than to overeat and feel bad or guilty about it later. Cutting out favorite snacks completely may cause upset that will result in later sabotage of your newly formed food behaviors.

SECTION 8

CURRENT NUTRITION TOPICS

SUGAR SUBSTITUTES

Many people are confronted with the use of sugar substitutes either to help with weight reduction or to reduce their sugar intake. The demand for low carbohydrate and low sugar foods has resulted in new sugar substitutes that have helped improve the flavor and textures of foods when used as sugar replacements. Some sugar substitutes have no influence on blood glucose levels, or they may have a small effect. Since foods containing sugar substitutes may have carbohydrate and calories, it is important to read labels to see what you are eating.

Sugar substitutes may allow consumption of sweets while reducing their carbohydrate and calorie levels. There have been some claims that sugar substitutes can increase a person's craving for sweets. There is currently no scientific evidence to support this claim.

There are two types of sugar substitutes: non-nutritive, containing no calories, and nutritive sweeteners, which do contain calories. Sugar substitutes are designated as GRAS (generally recognized as safe), or they are approved as food additives by the 1958 Food Additives Amendment to the Federal Food, Drug, and Cosmetic Act. Each sugar substitute is given an ADI (Acceptable Daily Intake). The ADI is determined by a review of all available safety and toxicological data on a given food additive. It is given as mg of the sweetener per kilogram body weight (mg/kg). Most consumers would have a very difficult time reaching an intake as high as the ADIs.

Non-nutritive sweeteners include: Acesulfame-K (Ace-K), Aspartame, Neotame, Saccharin, Sucralose, and Truvia. These sweeteners are known as intense sweeteners since foods require very little to sweeten the food. They are also non-cariogenic (do not cause dental cavities). None of the sweeteners below has any effect on blood glucose, cholesterol, or triglyceride levels.

- *Ace-K* is a stable sweetener 200 times sweeter than sugar. Ace-K can withstand high temperatures used in cooking and baking. The human body does not metabolize Ace-K and excretes it through the urine unchanged. Ace-K's ADI is 15 mg/kg body weight. It is found in over 4000 food products and is marketed with the names Sunette, Sweet One, and Sweet-n-Safe. It is safe for pregnant and nursing women, children, and persons with diabetes.
- *Aspartame* has been used as a tabletop sweetener since 1981 and has been added to foods and beverages since 1996. Aspartame is 200 times sweeter than sugar. It is absorbed into the bloodstream and used in normal body functions. Those individuals with phenylketonuria (PKU), a rare metabolic hereditary disease, need to limit their intake of phenylalanine and should not use aspartame. It has been extensively researched and is considered safe for pregnant and nursing women, children, and persons with diabetes. Aspartame has an ADI of 50 mg/kg body weight. Through the years, individuals have complained of numerous physical issues from using aspartame, including headache, dizziness, and seizures, but these claims have never been substantiated by research. Aspartame can be found under the brand names Equal, Nutrataste, Nutrasweet, and Instasweet. Aspartame is found in hot and cold beverages, cereals, gelatins, puddings, ice cream, yogurt, candy, gum, and pharmaceuticals. It is also sold in packets to sweeten food and drinks. Aspartame can be used in recipes, but when cooked for long periods of time, it loses its sweetness.
- *Neotame* is very similar to aspartame but is even sweeter. It is approximately 7,000-13,000 times sweeter than aspartame. It is partially absorbed by the small intestine and is rapidly metabolized. Only 20% of the phenylalanine is absorbed in the bloodstream so that individuals with PKU do not need to be cautioned with its use. Neotame can be used in baking, but with its intensive sweetness, it is blended with sugar to allow an acceptable product.
- *Saccharin* is the oldest approved sweetener and is 300 times sweeter than sugar. Saccharin can be combined with sugar for an acceptable sweetness. It has been used for over a century, and more than 30 studies have supported its safety. In 2000, the National Toxicology Program eliminated saccharin from its list of carcinogens. President Clinton signed

legislation to remove saccharin warning labels from foods, which had been in effect since 1977.

- *Sucralose* is the newest non-nutritive sweetener on the market and is 600 times sweeter than sugar. It is also heat-stable so it can be used for cooking. Over 20 years of research and testing have determined that sucralose is a safe product, and it has been approved by the FDA since 1999.

- *Truvia* is the new sweetener made from stevia. Japanese companies have been producing sweeteners extracted from this South American plant for decades. Cargill Company released the tabletop sweetener Truvia made from stevia in July 2008. Final FDA approval is needed before American companies can add this product to food products.

- *Polyols* are reduced-calorie sweeteners. They are not sugars or alcohols, but have a similar chemical structure to both sugar and alcohol. They are low-digestible carbohydrates used to replace sugar containing half the calories as sugar so that they provide fewer calories per gram than other carbohydrates. Polyols taste like sugar with a similar texture. They add bulk to products and a smooth texture to ice cream, fillings, frosting, yogurt, and fruit spreads. Polyols help with good oral health by decreasing tooth demineralization, plaque neutralization, and incidence of caries. They are also helpful in weight loss or weight maintenance and reduce overall glycemic load.

  When calculating the total carbohydrate from a food sweetened totally from polyols, foods with less than 10 grams of carbohydrate is considered a "free food". With greater than 10 grams of carbohydrate in a food, subtract half of the polyol grams from the total carbohydrate and then calculate the exchanges.

  Greater than 50 grams of polyols may cause gastrointestinal effects. These symptoms are usually mild and temporary. Individuals will generally adapt in a few days in the manner they would with an increase in fiber intake in the diet.

Often sweeteners are used in combination to improve taste and to improve the stability of the product. Consumers have also found that varying their use of sweeteners allows them to improve the taste and stability of products.

A new sweetener, altimame, is being filed for approval with the FDA. It is 2000 times sweeter than sugar and has good heat stability. Cyclamate reapproval is also being sought, although it is presently approved in over 50 countries. It is 30 times sweeter than sugar and when used with other sweeteners is acceptable.

The following chart is an example from www.caloriecontrol.org, that describes the approximate number of servings of different aspartame-containing products that an adult and child would need to consume to reach the ADI of 50mg/kg of body weight.

Aspartame –Containing Product	Approximate number of servings per day to reach the ADI	Approximate number of servings per day to reach the ADI
	Adult (150 lb.)	Child (50 lb.)
Carbonated soft drink (12 oz.)	20	6
Powdered soft drink (8 oz.)	33	11
Gelatin (4oz.)	42	14
Tabletop sweetener (packed)	97	32

Reprinted with permission from The Calorie Control Council

SUPERFOODS

"I'M STRONG TO THE FINISH WHEN I EATS MY SPINACH." -POPEYE

A superfood conjures up a vision of Popeye developing super strength after eating spinach. The popular media has grasped on to this idea with more than 40 items being identified as "superfoods."

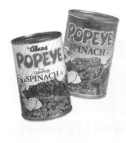

Superfoods are generally thought of as food items that are nutrient dense. They contain vitamins and/ or nutrients believed to contain special properties for disease prevention and/or longevity. Steven Pratt, MD, author of <u>Superfoods RX: Fourteen Foods That Will Change Your Life</u>, identifies the following foods to be extra "healthy" food items. These include:

FOOD	BENEFIT
Beans/Legumes	High in fiber, maintains healthy cholesterol and blood sugar levels.
Blueberries	Top source of antioxidants that protect the body against disease and may slow age-related brain decline, high fiber content maintains healthy cholesterol and blood sugar levels, and promotes a healthy immune response.
Oats	High in fiber, maintains healthy cholesterol and blood sugar levels.

FOOD	BENEFIT
Oranges	High source of Vitamin C that helps in maintaining a healthy heart, enhances immune function, and helps in fighting cancer with over 170 cancer-fighting phytochemicals and 60 flavinoids. Fights inflammation and works to promote healthy skin.
Pumpkin	High source of Vitamin A that promotes healthy skin, eyes, and immune function. Provides a good source of fiber that reduces cholesterol and smoothes out blood sugars. Good source of Vitamin C works to improve immune function.
Salmon	High in Omega-3 fatty acids that help in reducing heart disease, arthritis, aids in lowering cholesterol, and may help depression.
Soy	Helps to lower cholesterol levels, helps prevent heart disease, cancer, and osteoporosis.
Tea (green or black)	Contains potent antioxidants that help reduce allergies, fight heart disease and cancer, and slows the effects of aging.
Tomatoes	Contains the cancer-fighting antioxidant lycopene.
Turkey	One of the leanest sources of animal protein, low in cholesterol, fat and saturated fat. High in folic acid that protects against birth defects, some cancers, and heart disease.
Walnuts	High source of fiber, polypherols, vitamin E, Magnesium, protein, and Vitamin B6 that helps in maintaining a healthy heart and decreases risk of diabetes and cancer.
Yogurt	Contains probiotics that preliminary research suggest may help with digestive disorders, bacterial and yeast infections, food allergies, and immune function.
Dark Chocolate	Packed with antioxidants that preliminary research suggest may help in lowering blood pressure.

Although some foods are particularly high in certain nutrients, phytochemicals, and antioxidants, the Academy of Nutrition and Dietetics stresses eating a "super diet" rather than concentrating on a number of nutritionally dense foods. A super diet is one that follows the Dietary Guidelines for Americans that have been covered in this book. These guidelines along with consuming "superfoods," exercising regularly, and practicing healthy behaviors will help improve your health and reduce disease.

FOOD AND MOOD

"A GOOD LAUGH AND A LONG SLEEP ARE THE BEST CURES IN THE DOCTOR'S BOOK" – IRISH PROVERB

Who hasn't found comfort in a little chocolate, a bowl of ice cream, or a bag of chips? Using food for comfort, or during stressful times, is a problem that many of us struggle with during times of stress. Some say stress can be alleviated with the use of crunchy foods. Others find "creamy" or "smooth" foods produce calming or soothing effects. Turning to food when feeling blue can cause unwanted weight gain. Our patients who struggle with their weight state their emotions play a role in what they weigh. This additional weight can be caused not only by what you eat, but also by behaviors that cause you to eat.

WHAT WE EAT: NEUROTRANSMITTERS

Find yourself grumpy when on a low-carbohydrate diet? Scientists are now discovering a link between what we eat and how we feel. A study in the Archives of Internal Medicine investigated the effect on mood of a low carbohydrate diet (20 to 40 grams daily) equivalent to about 2 slices of bread or an apple and a slice of bread. The participants on the low-carb diet experienced more anxiety, anger, and depression than those on a low-fat, high carbohydrate diet. Carbohydrates promote serotonin, a chemical neurotransmitter in the brain that controls our mood, promoting good feelings.

Neurotransmitters, such as serotonin and norepinephrine, are involved in controlling mood and feeding behaviors. Neurotransmitters are substances that transmit nerve impulses. What we eat causes more, or less, of this transmission activity. For instance, unprocessed foods are found to contain more of the amino acids, or proteins, that create higher or lower levels of these neurotransmitters. Amino acids are proteins that are broken down in the body to form cells, hormones, and neurotransmitters, as well as performing other functions in the body. The British Journal of Psychiatry tracked 3,500 people eating a diet high in unprocessed, whole, foods such as fruits, vegetables, and unprocessed fresh meats. They found these people were less depressed than those with diets high in processed meats, refined foods, fried foods, and desserts.

Foods Containing Amino Acid Tryptophan	
Alfalfa sprouts	Eggs
Baked Beans	Endive
Beef	Fish
Broccoli	Milk
Brussels Sprouts	Soybeans
Carrots	Spinach
Cauliflower	Turkey
Celery	Turnips
Chicken	Watercress
Cottage Cheese	

Tryptophan is an amino acid which works to increase the serotonin level in the brain. Serotonin has been found to reduce moodiness, help with sleep, promote calmness, and stimulate the immune system. Tryptophan requires the presence of carbohydrates for entrance into the brain and to function appropriately. Diets with reduced carbohydrate intake cause a reduction in serotonin, which can increase moodiness.

Chocolate is often thought of as the ultimate comfort food. It contains the amino acid phenylalanine. This amino acid serves as a precursor for norepinephrine, which works in the brain as both an antidepressant and memory enhancer. Dark chocolate contains antioxidants (polyphenols) that researchers at Nestle Research Center in Switzerland found reduce stress hormones. Polyphenols are also found in fruits and vegetables. For this reason, some say that eating chocolate not only tastes delicious, but makes us smarter and feel better! Of course, there are other foods containing much fewer calories (dark chocolate is about 140 calories per ounce).

Foods Containing Amino Acid Phenylalanine	
Apples	Eggs
Avocados	Herring
Baked Beans	Milk
Bananas	Peanuts
Beef	Pineapple
Carrots	Soybeans
Chocolate	Spinach
Cottage Cheese	Tomatoes

Adding foods high in phenylalanine and tryptophan may be helpful in alleviating mild symptoms of depression, anxiety, and stress. If you find that certain foods cause negative mood changes, you should avoid them and discuss this with your physician and/or dietitian.

WHY WE EAT: STRESS AND BEHAVIORS

Feelings about food can build inappropriate behaviors, and over time, can cause us to consume the wrong types of foods, at the wrong times, and for the wrong reasons. If you find yourself gaining weigh during stressful times, you'll need to do some soul searching. Discover what triggers unwanted eating. Keep a log of foods (see chapter *Weighing Your Best* for help with how to log) and identify the feelings associated with overeating. Once you've discovered a connection between eating and your feelings, you'll need to "short circuit" the impulses driving you to eat. This can be accomplished by preselecting a few activities that you can "do" instead of eating.

Here are a few tips we suggest to our patients:

1. **Call a friend:** Catch up with a buddy you can talk with for at least 10 minutes.
2. **How hungry are you?** Sometimes we're really thirsty and the signal has been missed. Get a drink of water and wait 20 minutes before heading for food.
3. **Try and relax:** Take a few minutes for meditation.
4. **Take a short walk:** Around the block or around the office.
5. **Schedule meals and snacks:** Commit to not eating between meals except for planned snacks. Keep low calorie snacks available just in case an extra snack is necessary.
6. **Drink a no calorie beverage:** Something cold and refreshing in the summer and warm and soothing in the winter can curb your appetite.

Stop and think before you eat. Learn to ask yourself "how hungry am I?" and decide if it is an appropriate time to eat. Do you have some calories to spare? In other words try and remove the emotional component of eating.

CONCLUSION

So, here you are at the end of *Too Busy to Diet*. Perhaps you were just looking for some healthy menu ideas to add variety to your meals, or maybe you wanted to learn more about adding fiber or calcium to your diet. We hope *Too Busy to Diet* has served as a road map, helping you navigate the maze of eating situations that you face daily.

We've covered the nutrition topics that we think reflect the health concerns you might have. We believe the "Fav Five," weight, cholesterol, fiber, calcium, and exercise, are essential chapters for being healthy. Make sure to re-read them when you have a moment.

We know over the years you've been bombarded with nutrition information: TV and radio shows, web sites, magazines, books, and "wanna be nutritionists." In fact, there probably isn't a woman's magazine out there that doesn't supply us with nutrition information on a regular basis. Some is good information, some is not so good.

We hope we've provided the right information in just the right amount, enabling you to make the right choices. By now you may be shopping, reading food labels, and sitting down more often to a home cooked meal. Maybe you've even tried some delicious recipes that take less time to fix then stopping at a restaurant or waiting for carry out food. We hope so.

We think you'll find *Too Busy to Diet* is a great traveling companion or bedside reference. Our fundamental goal was to provide you with a guide that makes healthy living easy. We wish you healthy and happy eating.

APPENDIX A

FOOD DIARY

Daily Food Diary

Weight

Waist Circumference

Calorie Budget per Day

Day/Date	Time	Meal (B/L/D/Sn)	Food Record	Calories	Physical Activity	Mood

APPENDIX B

FOOD SAFETY

You may be questioning why a book for healthy people on the run would include a reference on food safety. A hectic lifestyle can make individuals more apt to forget food safety issues. How many busy people cannot remember when they brought leftovers home from a restaurant? How many of us forget to defrost meat for dinner and then put a package of meat on the counter to thaw? These practices can lead to a round of "Montezuma's Revenge" or plain old diarrhea or gastrointestinal upset.

The Centers for Disease Control & Prevention (CDC) reports that food poisoning is a great risk to Americans' safety. It has been estimated that approximately 76 million people get sick from food poisoning, 300,000 require hospitalization, and 5,000 Americans die each year from poor food safety practices. Not only do poor hygiene practices cause harm to our population, but we are spending a great deal of health care dollars on something that can be prevented. The Food and Drug Administration has placed the prevention of microbial contamination of the food supply as a high priority. But each one of us needs to do our job too.

The main causes of food borne Illness are bacteria, parasites, and viruses. They can be found in a wide variety of foods including dairy products, meat, spices, chocolate, seafood, and water.

There are specific foods that are implicated in food-borne illness. These include:
- Raw and undercooked eggs and foods containing undercooked eggs
- Chicken, tuna, potato, and macaroni salads
- Fresh produce
- Cream-filled pastries
- Unpasteurized fruit and vegetable juices and ciders

Bacteria have been found in raw seafood, and clams, cockles, mussels, oysters, and scallops may be contaminated with Hepatitis A. Improper food handling can cause the ideal environment for bacteria to grow. Common causes of poor food handling include:
- Hot or cold food left to stand too long at room temperature
- Improper cooking
- Using cutting boards and kitchen utensils to prepare contaminated food, such as raw chicken, and then using board for fruit or vegetables that will not be cooked.

Symptoms of food- borne Illness include:
- Abdominal Cramping
- Diarrhea
- Extreme Fatigue
- Fever
- Headache
- Vomiting
- Possible blood or pus in the stools

Generally the symptoms of food-borne illness vary depending on the amount of the contaminant eaten and the type of organism. Symptoms may occur as early as a half hour after eating the contaminated food. Typically symptoms do not develop for several days or weeks. Symptoms of viral or parasitic illnesses may take up to several weeks to develop. For the majority of persons, food-borne illness lasts for a day or two, but can last for 7-10 days. For healthy people, food-borne illness is not life-threatening and does not last long. Food-borne illness can be severe with:
- Babies and young children
- Elderly
- Alcoholism, viral hepatitis, and other liver diseases
- Diabetes
- Cancer
- Immune disorders
- HIV infection
- Gastrointestinal problems
- Steroid use for asthma and arthritis

Individuals with severe symptoms should see a doctor or seek emergency treatment. This is particularly important in those who are most vulnerable. Mild cases of food-borne illness should be treated with liquids to replace fluids lost from vomiting and diarrhea.

Food Safety Tips
There are many steps that can be taken to reduce the risk of food-borne illness. These include:
- Pick out packaged and canned foods first when shopping.
- Do not purchase cans that bulge or have dents.
- Avoid jars that are cracked or have loose or bulging lids.
- Do not eat raw shellfish and consume only pasteurized milk,

cheese, juices, and ciders if you are high risk.

- Buy eggs that are refrigerated, clean, and have no cracks.
- Purchase frozen foods and perishables such as meat, poultry, or fish last and place in separate bags to eliminate spillage of drippings on other food.
- Make sure that you buy meat or fish in stores that are clean and have a high customer base that insures fast turnover of items.
- Take an ice chest with you if it will take over an hour to get your groceries home to prevent spoilage of frozen or perishable foods.

Store Food Safely

- Refrigerate or freeze perishables promptly. Use a refrigerator/ freezer thermometer weekly to insure that the refrigerator is 40 degrees Fahrenheit (5 degrees Celsius) and the freezer is zero Fahrenheit (-18 degrees Celsius).
- Store leftovers in tight containers.
- Store eggs in their carton in the refrigerator and not on the door where the temperature is warmer.
- Keep seafood in the refrigerator or freezer until ready to prepare.
- Poultry and meat can be kept in plastic wrappers in the refrigerator for only a couple of days. Make sure the juices cannot escape to contaminate other foods.
- Do not crowd the refrigerator or freezer so that air cannot circulate.
- Moldy foods should be thrown out even though it is not a health threat, merely unappetizing. You may be able to save part of the moldy food by cutting out the mold and saving the remaining unaffected piece.
- Check labels on cans or jars for proper storage guidelines. Once a food has been opened it must be refrigerated. Examples include mayonnaise and ketchup.
- Do not thaw meat at room temperature. Move food from the freezer to the refrigerator for a day or two or defrost submerged in cold water. You can also defrost in the microwave. All defrosted foods must be used immediately.
- Do not eat foods that taste or smell funny. When in doubt, throw out.

Keep Your Kitchen Clean

- Wash hands with warm water and soap for 20 seconds before preparing food and after handling raw meat and poultry.

- Get rid of bacteria on counters with 1 teaspoon of chlorine bleach to 1 quart of water or with a kitchen cleaning agent diluted according to product directions.
- Keep dishcloths clean because they can harbor bacteria when wet. Wash dishcloths weekly in hot water in the washing machine.
- Sanitize the kitchen sink with 1 teaspoon bleach to 1 quart of water or use a kitchen cleaning agent. Food particles trapped in the drain and disposal are an ideal place for bacterial growth.
- Use cutting boards that are smooth, non-porous, and made of hard maple or plastic. They should be free of cracks and crevices. Use a scrub to clean with hot water and soap. Sanitize by rinsing in a solution of 1 tsp. chlorine bleach to 1 quart water or sanitize in the dishwasher.
- Wash and sanitize cutting boards used for raw foods, like seafood or chicken. Or use a separate cutting board for raw foods.
- Use clean utensils or wash utensils between the cutting of different foods.
- Clean lids of canned foods before opening to eliminate dirt from contaminating the food.
- Clean the can opener blade after each use. Food processers and meat grinders must be cleaned immediately after use.
- Do not place cooked meat in an unwashed plate or platter that has held raw meat.
- Wash fruits and vegetables thoroughly under running water. Use a small brush to remove surface dirt. Do not use soap or other detergents.

Watch Food Temperatures

Always keep hot food hot and cold foods cold. Check the Safe Minimum Cooking Temperatures and Food Storage Periods to insure food safety. For more complete food safety information check the website: www. Foodsafety.gov.

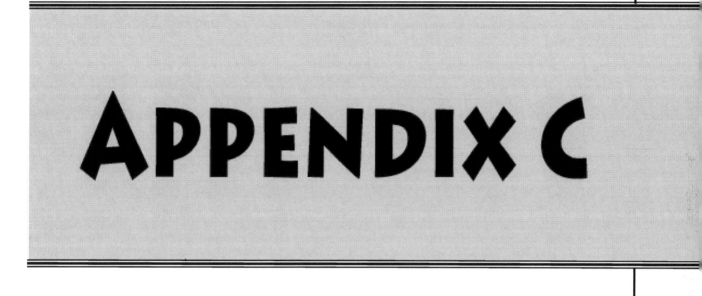

APPENDIX C

MEAL PLANS

Breakfast Meal plans

Meal plans were developed showing the food components that should be included daily for good nutrition. The below symbols represent these food components. Please note that some of the meals may be missing some of the food components. This accounts for days when you are in a rush or are saving your food for a holiday meal or a larger meal out. It is encouraged that you attempt to eat all of the food components at each meal when you can. Make up for missed foods at snacks or save for a larger meal later in the day when needed.

High Fiber   F
Heart Healthy   ♥
Calcium Rich   C

(1) 1 small whole wheat bagel F ♥ 1 slice 2% cheese slice C 1/3 cantaloupe F ♥ 1 cup skim milk ♥ C 1 cup blueberries F ♥	(2) 2 low-fat, whole wheat waffles F ♥ 1 tbs. lite syrup 2 tsp. soft tub margarine ♥ 1 ¼ cups fresh strawberries F ♥ 1 cup skim milk ♥ C	(3) 1 cup 80-100-calorie, low-fat yogurt C ♥ ¼ cup low fat granola F ♥ 1 slice whole wheat toast F ♥ 1 tsp. soft tub margarine ♥ Small fresh orange F ♥
(4) 1 ½ cups Cheerios F ♥ 1 slice whole wheat toast F ♥ 1 tsp. soft tub margarine ♥ Small banana F ♥ 1 cup skim milk ♥ C	(5) 1 cup cooked oatmeal F ♥ 2 tbs. raisins F ♥ 1 cup skim milk ♥ C	(6) Large whole wheat bagel F ♥ 1 tbs. lite cream cheese (4 ounces) 1 cup skim milk or 100-calorie yogurt ♥ C
(7) 1 slice leftover thin cheese pizza C Small fresh apple F ♥	(8) Granola bar F ♥ 1 cup 100-calorie yogurt F ♥ 17 grapes F ♥	(9) ¼ cup low-fat cottage cheese C 1 unsweetened pineapple half F ♥ 2 slices raisin toast F ♥ 2 tsp. soft tub margarine ♥
(10) Whole wheat English muffin F ♥ 1 tbs. peanut butter ♥ Small fresh peach F ♥ 1 cup skim milk ♥ C	(11) Cupcake-size low-fat bran muffin F ♥ 1 tsp. soft tub margarine ♥ 1 cup 100-calorie, low-fat yogurt ♥ C F Small fresh pear F ♥	(12) 2 slices whole wheat toast F ♥ 1 scrambled egg with 1 slice 2% fat cheese C 2 tsp. soft tub margarine ♥ half grapefruit F ♥

(13)	(14)	(15)
2 slices French whole wheat toast F ♥ 2 tsp. soft tub margarine ♥ 1 tbs. lite syrup 1 cup 100-calorie, low-fat yogurt ♥ C small fresh banana F ♥	2 medium whole wheat pancakes F ♥ 1 tbs. lite syrup 1 cup blueberries F ♥ 1 cup skim milk ♥ C	Cheese omelet (made with 1 egg white and 2 egg whites): 2% fat cheese (1 slice) C 1 egg and 2 egg whites 2 slices whole wheat toast F ♥ 1 orange F ♥
(16)	(17)	(18)
Whole wheat English muffin F ♥ 1 slice 2% fat cheese C 1 fresh apple F ♥	Breakfast burrito: 1 scrambled egg 1 whole wheat tortilla F ♥ 1 slice 2% fat cheese salsa Fresh fruit cup F ♥	1 hard-boiled egg Granola bar F ♥ 100-calorie, low-fat yogurt ♥ C Small banana F ♥
(19)	(20)	(21)
3 graham cracker squares F ♥ 2 tbsp peanut butter ♥ 1 cup skim milk ♥ C Tangerine F ♥	1 whole wheat English muffin F ♥ 1 ounce slice lean ham ♥ 2 light pineapple rings 1 cup skim milk ♥ C	Thomas 100-calorie whole wheat English muffin F ♥ 2 tsp soft tub margarine ♥ 1 cup 100-calorie, low- fat yogurt ♥ C 1 small banana F ♥
(22)	(23)	(24)
Thomas 100-calorie whole wheat bagel F ♥ 2 tsp soft tub margarine ♥ 1 cup 100-calorie low –fat yogurt ♥ C 1 small pear F ♥	½ cup trail mix F ♥ 1 cup 100-calorie, low-fat yogurt ♥ C	1 cup 100-calorie, low- fat yogurt ♥ C ¼ cup grape nuts F ♥ 1 small banana F ♥
(25)	(26)	(27)
Peanut butter and Jelly toast: 1 tbsp peanut butter ♥ 1 tsp all-fruit jelly 2 slices whole wheat toast F ♥ 1 cup skim milk ♥ C 1 ¼ c. Strawberries F ♥	1 whole wheat pita F ♥ ¼ cup low-fat cottage cheese C 1 small banana sliced F ♥	Granola F ♥ Yogurt ♥ C Mixed berries F ♥
(28)	(29)	(30)
Fresh fruit kabob (can include: strawberries, grapes, blueberries, and other fresh fruits of your liking) F ♥ 1 Cranberry Orange low-fat muffin F ♥ Skim milk ♥ C	Lox with cucumbers, sliced tomatoes, on mixed greens F ♥ Small whole wheat bagel F ♥ Low-fat cream cheese C Fresh Grapes and Strawberries F ♥ Skim milk ♥ C	Breakfast Quesadilla: Whole wheat tortilla F ♥ Fresh Fruit cup F ♥ 1 slice 2% fat cheddar cheese C

Lunch Meal Plans

Vegetarian Choices are marked in parenthesis to allow the entire family to eat the same base meal with the vegetarian alternate provided for the vegetarian member.

High Fiber   F
Heart Healthy   ♥
Calcium Rich   C

(1)	(2)	(3)
2-4ounces grilled salmon ♥ Mixed greens F ♥ (Hard cooked egg and cheese slices) or feta cheese C 2 tbs. lite salad dressing ♥ Large whole wheat roll F ♥ Large apple F ♥	2 small soft whole wheat tortillas F ♥ 2-4 ounces grilled chicken ♥ (Black beans) F ♥ (1 ounce grated 2 % cheese) C Lettuce/tomato F ♥ Large orange F ♥	2 slices whole wheat bread F ♥ 2-4 ounces turkey ♥ (Scrambled eggs) Lettuce/tomato F ♥ Large pear F ♥
(4)	(5)	(6)
2-4 ounces water-packed tuna ♥ (2 slices 2 % cheese) C 2 slices whole wheat bread F ♥ 1 tsp. lite mayonnaise ♥ Lettuce/tomato F ♥ Raw carrots F ♥ Large peach F ♥	1 cup vegetable soup F ♥ 6 whole wheat crackers F ♥ 2 slices 2% fat cheese C 34 grapes F ♥	2 slices whole wheat bread F ♥ 2 tbs. peanut butter ♥ 1 tsp. no-sugar jelly 1 ¼ cups strawberry F ♥
(7)	(8)	(9)
1 cup homemade chili made with lean beef or turkey F ♥ (Vegetarian chili) F ♥ 1 ounce grated cheese C	Frozen luncheon meal (Frozen vegetarian meal) Salad F ♥ 2 tbs. lite salad dressing ♥ Slice of whole wheat bread F ♥ 2 small tangerines F ♥	Vegetable omelet F ♥ 2 slices whole wheat toast F ♥ 2 tsp. lite margarine ♥ Fresh fruit cup F ♥
(10)	(11)	(12)
1 cup chicken noodle soup 6 whole wheat crackers F ♥ 1 slice 2% fat cheese C Small plum F ♥	60-90 calorie yogurt ♥ C Fresh apple F ♥ 2 tbs. peanut butter ♥ Small low-fat muffin ♥ 1 tsp. lite margarine ♥	2-4 ounces grilled chicken ♥ (Hard cooked egg and 2 ounces 2% cheese) Mixed greens F ♥ 2 tbs. lite salad dressing ♥ 2 large bread sticks 1 cup diet applesauce F ♥
(13)	(14)	(15)
2-4 ounces grilled fish ♥ (2/3 cup brown rice) (2/3 cup kidney beans) Steamed broccoli Salad 2 tbs. lite salad dressing ♥ Fresh pear	Low calorie lunch 100 calorie whole wheat English muffin 2 slices 50 calorie cheese Large fresh fruit	Low calorie Lunch 50 calorie high fiber tortilla (2)50 calorie 2% cheese slices or turkey slices Large fresh fruit

(16) Lunch on the run: Slim fast or Carnation Instant Breakfast C Fresh Fruit F ♥ 1 starch—pretzels, roll, crackers	(17) Leftover manicotti, lasagna C Salad F ♥ 2 tbs. lite dressing ♥ Fresh orange F ♥	(18) Trail Mix F ♥ (300 calorie portion) 100 calorie, low-fat yogurt ♥ C
(19) 2 ounces peanut butter pretzels Fresh fruit F ♥	(20) 100 calorie, low-fat yogurt ♥ C Fresh fruit F ♥ Whole wheat roll F ♥	(21) 2 Mozzarella sticks C Fresh fruit F ♥ Whole wheat Crackers F ♥
(22) Energy bar with at least 10 grams protein Fresh fruit F ♥	(23) Macaroni and cheese C Salad F ♥ 2 tbs. lite dressing ♥ Fresh Peach F ♥	(24) Egg salad Hard-cooked eggs Low fat mayonnaise ♥ Celery F ♥ High fiber tortilla F ♥ Fresh pear F ♥
(25) Hummus F ♥ Lettuce and Tomato F ♥ Whole wheat tortilla F ♥ Fresh grapes F ♥	(26) Chicken salad Chopped chicken ♥ Low-fat mayonnaise ♥ Celery F ♥ Whole wheat toast F ♥ Fresh plums F ♥	(27) Chicken Strips ♥ Mixed Baby Greens F ♥ Oil and vinegar ♥ Whole wheat roll F ♥ Margarine ♥ Fresh orange F ♥
(28) Roasted turkey roll ♥ Low fat Cole slaw ♥ Spinach tortilla F ♥ Fresh orange F ♥		

Dinner Meal Plans

Vegetarian Choices are marked in parenthesis to allow the entire family to eat the same base meal with the vegetarian alternate provided for the vegetarian member.

High Fiber   F

Heart Healthy   ♥

Calcium Rich   C

(1) Frozen dinner meal (vegetarian frozen meal) Salad with tomatoes, raw vegetables F ♥ 1 tsp. olive oil and vinegar Small whole wheat roll F ♥ 1 ¼ cup fresh strawberries F ♥	(2) Grilled chicken breast ♥ (2/3 cup kidney, black, or garbanzo beans) F ♥ (2/3 cup brown rice) F ♥ ½ cup green beans F ♥ (fresh salad) F ♥ 2 tbs. lite salad dressing ♥ Fresh apple F ♥	(3) Baked orange roughy ♥ (2 % fat grated cheese) C Large baked potato with skin F ♥ 2 tbs. lite sour cream C Broccoli F ♥ Fresh orange F ♥
(4) Pork tenderloin ♥ (Tofu) ♥ Stir-fry vegetables F ♥ 1 cup whole wheat pasta F ♥ fresh salad F ♥ 2 tbs. lite salad dressing ♥ Fresh blueberries (1 cup) F ♥	(5) Lean hamburger ♥ (Veggie burger) ♥ Hamburger bun Lettuce/tomato F ♥ ½ cup mushrooms F ♥ Fresh grapes F ♥	(6) 3 ounces imitation crab meat (2 ounce 2 % fat cheese) C 2 small spinach tortillas F ♥ Tomato F ♥ Lettuce F ♥ Salad F ♥ 2 tbs. lite salad dressing ♥ ½ cup mandarin oranges F ♥
(7) Lamb chop ♥ (chicken textured protein) ♥ (grilled portobello mushroom) F ♥ 1 cup whip potatoes ½ cup carrots F ♥ Salad F ♥ 2 tbs. lite salad dressing ♥ Fresh watermelon F ♥	(8) Vegetable omelet 2 slices whole wheat toast F ♥ 2 tsp. lite margarine ♥ Fresh cantaloupe F ♥	(9) 2 slices whole wheat toast F ♥ 2-4 ounces tuna ♥ (2 slices 2 % cheese slices) C Lite mayonnaise ♥ Raw celery sticks F ♥ Fresh peach F ♥
(10) 1 ½ cups whole wheat pasta F ♥ Lean meat sauce (tomato sauce) 2 tbs. parmesan cheese C Large mixed salad F ♥ 2 tbs. lite salad dressing ♥ Large banana F ♥	(11) 2 small soft whole wheat tortillas F ♥ 2-3 ounces grilled chicken or lean turkey or beef ♥ (2/3 cup kidney, garbanzo, or black beans) ♥ 1 ounce 2% fat grated cheese C Lettuce/ tomatoes F ♥ Large Apple F ♥	(12) Large baked potato with skin F ♥ 2-4 ounces 2% fat cheese C Broccoli F ♥ 2 tbs. lite sour cream Salad F ♥ 2 tbs. lite salad dressing ♥ 1 ounce 2% fat grated cheese C Large fresh pear F ♥
(13) 2 slices thin sliced cheese or vegetable pizza C Fresh salad F ♥ 2 tbs. lite salad dressing ♥ ½ cup fruit cup F ♥	(14) Grilled cheese sandwich: (made with 2% fat cheese, lite- margarine, 2 slices whole wheat bread) C F ♥ 1 cup vegetable soup F ♥ ½ cup natural applesauce F ♥	(15) Pork chop (Tofu) ♥ 2/3 cup brown rice F ♥ Pineapple slices/green peppers F ♥ Salad F ♥ 2 tbs. lite salad dressing ♥

(16) 4 ounces steak (Veggie Burger) ½ cup green beans F ♥ Baked potato with skin F ♥ 1 tbs. lite sour cream ♥ Salad 2 tbs. lite salad dressing ♥ Fresh small banana	**(17)** Chicken roll-up with 3 ounces chicken slices ♥ (kidney, garbanzo, or black beans) ♥ 1 ounce grated 2% fat cheese C Lettuce F ♥ Light mayonnaise ♥ Salad F ♥ 1 tsp. olive oil and vinegar ♥ ½ mango F ♥	**(18)** Grilled tuna sandwich on a whole wheat bun or W.W. English muffin F ♥ (Grilled Eggplant) F ♥ (1 ounce mozzarella cheese) C Raw carrots and celery F ♥ Large fresh Apple F ♥
(19) 1 cup whole wheat spaghetti F ♥ Chicken strips ♥ (marinara sauce) Salad F ♥ 1 tsp. olive oil and vinegar ♥ Small peach F ♥	**(20)** 4 ounces grilled salmon ♥ (kidney, garbanzo, or black beans) ♥ (shrimp) (tempeh or seitan) Broccoli F ♥ 1 cup brown rice F ♥ Salad F ♥ 2 tbs. lite salad dressing ♥ 2 small plums F ♥	**(21)** 1 cup meat chili F ♥ (1 cup vegetarian chili with beans) F ♥ 1 ounce 2% fat cheese C Salad F ♥ 2 tbs. lite salad dressing ♥ Small orange F ♥
(22) Pork stir-fry ♥ (tofu or vegetable stir-fry) F ♥ Sugar snap peas F ♥ 1 cup brown rice F ♥ Salad F ♥ 2tbs. lite salad dressing ♥ 1 cup blueberries F ♥	**(23)** ½ cup chili beans F ♥ 1 ounce 2% fat grated cheese C 2 small whole wheat tortillas F ♥ Salad F ♥ 1 tsp. olive oil and vinegar ♥ Small orange F ♥	**(24)** 4 ounces Tilapia ♥ (lentils) F ♥ 1 cup couscous F ♥ Broccoli ♥ Salad F ♥ 2 tbs. lite salad dressing ♥ 1/3 cantaloupe F ♥
(25) Frozen cheese ravioli C Tomato sauce Salad F ♥ 2 tbs. lite salad dressing ♥ 1 ¼ cup strawberries F ♥	**(26)** Roast turkey ♥ (Butternut or spaghetti squash) F ♥ 1 cup stuffing Salad F ♥ 1 tsp. olive oil and vinegar ♥ Small peach F ♥	**(27)** Round steak ♥ (veggie sausage or soyrizo) ♥ Green peppers F ♥ 1 cup brown rice F ♥ Salad F ♥ 2 tbs. salad dressing ♥ 1 cup watermelon F ♥
(28) Roasted turkey roll ♥ Low fat Cole slaw ♥ Spinach tortilla F ♥ Fresh orange F ♥	**(29)** Hearty bean soup F ♥ French bread Salad F ♥ 2 tbs. lite salad dressing ♥ 1 cup fruit salad F ♥	**(30)** Vegetable lasagna C Salad F ♥ 2 tbs. lite dressing ♥ Small apple F ♥
(31) Gnocchi Meat sauce (Marina sauce) Salad F ♥ 2 tbs. lite dressing ♥ 1 cup berries F ♥	**(32)** Cheese quesadillas C Lettuce and tomato F ♥ Vegetable soup F ♥ 1/3 cantaloupe F ♥	**(33)** ½ cup no fat Cottage cheese ♥ Whole wheat roll F ♥ 1 tsp. lite margarine ♥ 1 cup fruit cocktail F ♥

(34) Peanut butter sandwich on whole wheat bread F ♥ Raw celery sticks F ♥ 1/3 honeydew melon F ♥	(35) Macaroni and cheese C Fresh salad F ♥ 2 tbs. lite dressing ♥ Small apple F ♥	

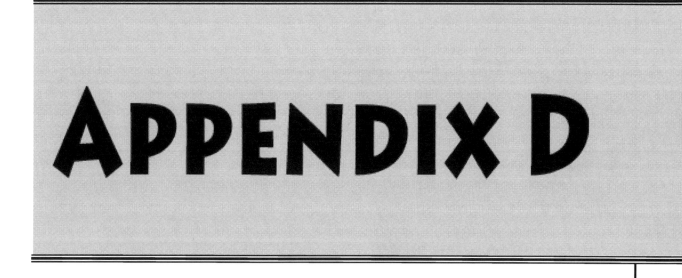

APPENDIX D

SUGGESTED RESOURCES

Suggested Books

1. Price, Jessie
   The Simple Art of Eating Well Test Kitchen
   Eating Well Test Kitchen

2. Hornick, Betsy & Chamberlain, Richard
   The Healthy Beef Cookbook
   National Cattlemen's Beef Association
   John Wiley & Sons, 2006

3. Napier, Kristine & Food and Culinary Professionals
   American Dietetic Association Cooking Healthy Across America
   American Dietetic Association
   John Wiley & Sons, 2004

4. Duyff, Roberta Larson, MS, RD, FADA, CFS
   365 Days of Healthy Eating from the American Dietetic Association
   John Wiley & Sons, 2003

5. Castle, Stacie, RD; Cotler, Robyn, RD; Scheftner, Marni, RD; Shapiro, Shana, RD
   Bite it & Write It: A Guide to Keeping Track of What You Eat & Drink
   Square One Publishing, 2011

6. Lindberg, Alexander, MD
   Eating the Greek Way
   Clarkson Potter Publications, 2007

7. Ponichtera ,Brenda J.,RD
   Quick and Healthy Recipes and Ideas
   Small Steps Press,2008

8. Ponichtera, Brenda J., RD
   Quick and Healthy Volume II
   Small Steps Press, 2009

9. Nelson, Miriam E., PhD.
   Strong Women Stay Young
   Bantam Book, 2005

10. Rondinielli, Lara, RD, CDE & Bucko, Jennifer
   Healthy Eating Calendar Diabetic Cooking
   American Diabetes Association, 2004

11. Borushek, Allan
   Calorie King Calorie, Fat, and Carbohydrate Counter 2012
   www.calorieking.com

12. Davis, Brenda, RD & Melinda, Vesanto, MS, RD with Berry, Ryan
   Becoming Raw: The Essential Guide to Raw Vegan Diets

13. Adle, Karen & Fertig, Judith
   The Gardner & the Grill: The Bounty of the Garden Meets the Sizzle of the Grill

Suggested Applications

1. CalorieCount.com
2. LoseIt.com
3. WebMD.com Food and Fitness Planner
4. MyFitnessPal.com
5. SparkPeople.com
6. EatingWell.com/menuplanner
7. MealSnap.com
8. Whole Foods Market app
9. AllRecipes.com Dinner Spinner
10. Kelloggsnutrition.com/fiber-tracker-mobile/
11. Calorieking.com

Suggested Magazines

1. www.CleanEating.com
2. www.EatingWell.com
3. www.CookingLight.com
4. www.diabeticlivingonline.com

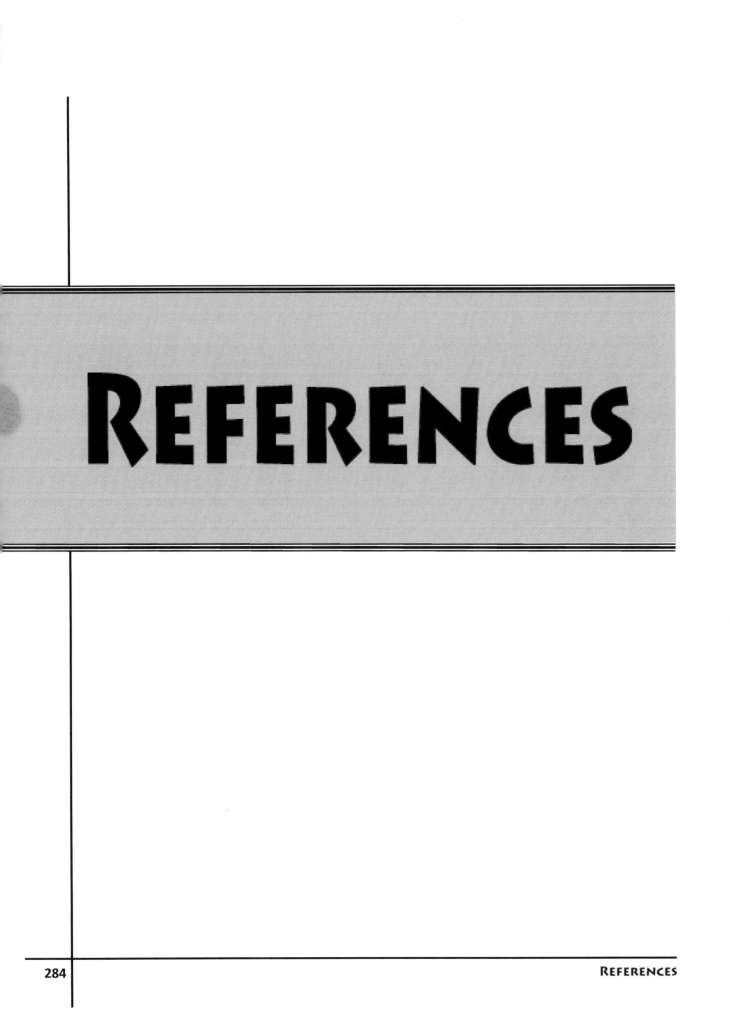

REFERENCES

1. Alexandria D Blatt, Liane S Roe, and Barbara J Rolls, Hidden vegetables: An effective Strategy to reduce energy intake and increase vegetable intake in adults, American Journal of Clinical Nutrition, February 2011,95 (2).

2. American Beverage Association (ABA), http://www.ameribev.org

3. American Dietetic Association Position Statement on Superfoods Neuhouser ML, Wassertheil-Smoller S, Thomson C *et al.* (2009). "Multivitamin use and risk of cancer and cardiovascular disease in the Women's Health Initiative cohorts". *Arch Internal Medicine, vol.169 No.3, February 9, 2009.*

4. American Heart Association (AHA), Statement On Caffeine. (2007). http://www.americanheart.org/presenter.jhtml

5. American Heart Association. Carbohydrates and Sugars. Accessed April 20, 2010. http://www.americanheart.org/presenter

6. Andersen, L.F., Jacobs, D.R, Jr, Carlsen, M.H., Blomhoff, Rune. Consumption of coffee is associated with reduced risk of death attributed to inflammatory and cardiovascular diseases in the Iowa Women's Health Study. *Am. J. Clinical Nutrition,* May 2006; 83: 1039.

7. Berni C. Ruotolo S., Discepolo V, Troncone R. The diagnosis of food allergy in children. Curr Opin Pediatr. 2008; 20(5):584-9.

8. Bischoff-Ferrari HA, Willett WC, Wong JB, Giovannucci E, Dietrich T, Dawson-Hughes B. Fracture prevention with vitamin D supplementation: a meta-analysis of randomized controlled trials. *JAMA.* 2005; 293:2257-64.

9. Boonen S, Lips P, Bouillon R, Bischoff-Ferrari HA, Vanderschueren D, Haentjens P. Need for additional calcium to reduce the risk of hip fracture with vitamin D supplementation: evidence from a comparative meta-analysis of randomized controlled trials. *J Clin Endocrinol Metab.* 2007; 92:1415-23.

10. Cnattingius, S., Signorello, L.B., Anneren, G., Clausson, B., Ekbom, A., Ljunger, E., Blot, W.J., McLaughlin, J.K., Petersson, G., Rane, A., Granath, F. Caffeine intake and the risk of first-trimester spontaneous abortion. *N Eng J Med.* 2000; Dec 21; 343(25):1839-1845.

11. Community gardening; Wikipedia, en.wikipedia.orgwiki/ Community_gardening

12. Diabetes Care, March 2008, vol 31,no.3, 596-615. Economic Costs of Diabetes in the U.S. in 2007.

13. Dietary Reference Intakes: Food and Nutrition Board of Institute of Medicine National Academy Press, Wash. D.C., 7/29/2011.

14. Dr. Kevin D Hall PhD, Gary Sachs PhD, Dhruva Chandramohen BSc, Car-

son C Chow PhD, Y Claire Wang MD, Steven L Gortmaker PhD, Boyd A. Swinburn MD. The Lancet Volume 378, Issue 9793, pages 826-837, August 2011.

15. Environmental Working Group. Sugar in Children's Cereals, http://ww.ewg.org/report/sugar-in-children's-Cereals/more_sugar-25K

16. Essential Guide to Vitamins and Minerals: Second Edition, Revised and Updated by Elizabeth Somer, Health Media of America, 1/14, 96. Harper Collins Publishers, 10East 53rd St., New York, New York 10022.

17. Francois-Pierre J. Martin, Serge Rezzi, Emma Per-Trepat, Beate Kamlage, Sebastiano Collino, Edgar Leibold, Jrgen Kastler, Dietrich Rein, Laurent B. Fay and Sunil Kochhar.Metabolic Effects of Dark Chocolate Consumption on Energy, Gut Microbiota, and Stress-Related Metabolism in Free-Living Subjects,*Journal of Proteome Research*, 2009.

18. Good CK, Holschuh NM, Albertson AM, Eldridge AL. whole grain consumption and body mass index in adult women: an analysis of NHANES 1999-2000 and the USDA Pyramid Serving Database. J Am Cull Nutr 2008; 27:80-7.

19. Gorin AA, Phelan S, Hill JO, Wing RR. (2004). Medical triggers are associated with better short- and long-term weight loss outcomes. *Preventive Medicine*, 39, 612-16.

20. Gorin AA, Phelan S, Wing RR, Hill JO. (2004). Promoting long-term weight control: does dieting consistency matter? *International Journal of Obesity and Related Metabolic Disorders*, 28, 278-81.

21. Grant D. Brinkworth, PhD; Jonathan D. Buckley, PhD; Manny Noakes, PhD; Peter M. Clifton, PhD; Carlene J. Wilson, PhD, Long-term Effects of a Very Low-Carbohydrate Diet and a Low-Fat Diet on Mood and Cognitive Function, *Arch Intern Med.* 2009; 169(20):1873-1880.

22. Hamnid R., Farshchi, Moira A.Tayhlor, and Ian Mac Donald., Increased LDI levels Deleterious Effects of Omitting Breakfast on insulin sensitivity and fasting lipids, American Journal of Clinical Nutrition, February 2005 vol 81(2)388-396.

23. Holick MF. Vitamin D deficiency. *N Engl J Med.* 2007; 357:266-81.

24. Holick MF. Vitamin D: importance in the prevention of cancers, type 1 diabetes, heart disease, and osteoporosis. *Am J Clin Nutr.* 2004; 79:362-71.

25. Holt, SH, Miller, JC, Petocz, D, Farmakalidis E. Department of Biochemistry University of Sydney, Australia: A Satiety Index of Common Foods, European Journal of Clinical Nutrition, 1995 Sept; 49 (9): 675-90.

26. Holt, SH, Miller, JC, Petocz, D, Farmakalidis E. Department of Biochemistry University of Sydney, Australia: A Satiety Index of Common Foods, European Journal of Clinical Nutrition, 1995 Sept;49 (9): 675-90

27. I-min Lee, Luc Djousse, et.al, JAMA, 2010; 303(12) 1173-1179.Physical Activity and Weight Gain Prevention.

28. Institute of Medicine. *Dietary Reference Intakes for Calcium and Vitamin D.* Washington, D.C.: National Academies Press, 2010.

29. Iris Shal, R.D.Ph.D, Dan Schwarzfuchs, M.D., Yaakov Henkin, M.D. Danit R. Sshahar, R.D., Ph.D., Shula Witkow, R.d., M.P.H., Liana Greenberg, R.D., M.P.H., Rachel Golan, R.D., M.P.H., Drora Fraser, Ph.D., Arkady Bolotin, Ph.D, Hilel Vardi, M.Sc., Osnat Tangi-Rozental, B.A. Rachel Zuk-Ramot, R.N., Benjamin Sarusi, M.Sc., Dov Brickner, M.D., Ziva Fiedler, M.D. Matthias Bluher, M.d. Michael Stumvoll, M.D. and Meir J. Stampfer, M.D., Dr.P.H. for the dietary Intervention Randomized Controlled Trial (DIRECT) Group Weight Loss with a Low-Carbohydrate, Mediterranean , or Low-Fat Diet: New Engl J Med 2008; 359:229-241, July 2008.

30. Jensen, MK, Koh-Baneijee P, Hu FB, Franz, M Sampson, L, Gronbaek M, Rimm EB, Intakes of Whole grains, Beans and Grain and the Risk of Coronary Heart Disease in Men. American Journal of clinical Nutrition 2004 Decl80 (6): 1492-9.

31. Johnson RK, Frary C. "Choose beverages and foods to moderate your intake of sugars: the 2000 dietary guidelines for Americans--what's all the fuss about?" J Nutr. 2001 Oct;131(10):2766S-2771S.

32. Journal of the American Medical Association. "Caloric Sweetener Consumption and Dyslipidemia Among US Adults." Accessed April 20, 2010.

33. Katzmanzyk, PT, Church, TS, Craig, C L, and Bouchard,C. (2009). Sitting time and mortality from all causes cardiovascular disease and cancer. Medicine and Science in Sports and Exercise, 2009 May ;41 (5), 998-100.

34. Kevin D Hall PhD, Gary Sachs PhD, Dhruva Chandramohen BSc, Carson C Chow PhD, Y Claire Wang MD, Steven L Gortmaker PhD, Boyd A. Swinburn MD, The Lancet Volume 378, Issue 9793, pages 826-837, August 2011.

35. Klem ML, Wing RR, Chang CH, Lang W, McGuire MT, Sugerman HJ, Hutchison SL, Makovich AL & Hill JO. (2000). A case-control study of successful maintenance of a substantial weight loss: Individuals who lost weight through surgery versus those who lost weight through non-surgical means. *International Journal of Obesity*, 24, 573-579.

36. Klem ML, Wing RR, McGuire MT, Seagle HM & Hill JO (1997). A descriptive study of individuals successful at long-term maintenance of substantial weight loss. *American Journal of Clinical Nutrition*, 66, 239-246.

37. Klem ML, Wing RR, McGuire MT, Seagle HM & Hill JO. (1998). Psychological symptoms in individuals successful at long-term maintenance of weight loss. *Health Psychology*, 17, 336-345.

38. Klem ML, Wing, RR, Lang W, McGuire MT & Hill JO. (2000). Does weight loss maintenance become easier over time? *Obesity Research*, 8, 438-444.

39. Lee I, Djoussé L, Sesso HD, Wang L, Buring JE. Physical activity and weight gain prevention. JAMA. 2010;303(12):1173-1179.

40. Liu, S, Willett WC, Manson JE, Hu FB, Rosner B, Colditz G. Relation between changes in intakes of dietary fiber and grain products and changes in weight and development of obesity among middle-aged women. Am J Clin Nutr 2003;78:920-7.

41. Marge Condrasky, Jenny Ledke, Julie E.Flood, Barbara J.Rolls, Chefs Opinion of Restaurant Portion Sizes. Obesity (2007) 15, 2086-2094.

42. McGuire MT, Wing RR, Hill JO. (1999). The prevalence of weight loss maintenance among American adults. *International Journal of Obesity*, 23, 1314 -1319.

43. McGuire MT, Wing RR, Klem ML, Hill JO (1999). The Behavioral characteristics of individuals who lose weight unintentionally. *Obesity Research*, 7, 485-490.

44. McGuire MT, Wing RR, Klem ML, Hill JO. (1999). Behavioral strategies of individuals who have maintained long-term weight losses. *Obesity Research*, 7, 334-341.

45. McGuire MT, Wing RR, Klem ML, Lang W & Hill JO. (1999). What predicts weight regain among a group of successful weight losers? *Journal of Consulting & Clinical Psychology*, 67, 177-185.

46. McGuire MT, Wing RR, Klem ML, Seagle HM & Hill JO (1998). Long-term maintenance of weight loss: Do people who lose weight through various weight loss methods use different behaviors to maintain their weight? *International Journal of Obesity*, 22, 572-577.

47. McKeown NM. Yoshida M, Shea MK, Jacques PF, Lichtenstein AH, Rogers G, Booth SL, Saltzman E. Whole-grain intake and cereal fiber are associated with lower abdominal adiposity in older adults. J Nutr 2009;139;1950 -5.

48. Neuhouser ML, Wassertheil-Smoller S, Thomson C *et al.* (2009). "Multivitamin use and risk of cancer and cardiovascular disease in the Women's Health Initiative cohorts". *Arch Internal Medicine, vol.169 No.3, February 9, 2009.*

49. Neumark-Sztainer, D.M.Wall, J.Guo, M. Story, J Haines, and M.Eisenhberg. 2006 Obesity, Disordered eating, and eating disorders in a longitudinal study of adolescents: How dieters fare five years later? J Amer Diet Assoc 106: 44)559-568.

50. Oldways' Mediterranean Diet Pyramid. (2009). Retrieved from, www.oldwayspt.org

51. Phelan S, Wing RR, Hill JO, Dibello J. (2003). Recovery from relapse among successful weight maintainers. *American Journal of Clinical Nutrition*, 78, 1079-1084.

52. Raynor H, Wing RR, Phelan S. (2005). Amount of food group variety consumed in the diet and long-term weight loss maintenance. *Obesity Research*, 13, 883-890.

53. Rideout TC, Lun B. Plant Sterols in the Management of Dyslipidemia in Patients with Diabetes. On the Cutting Edge. 2010;31(6):13-17.

54. *Rolls BJ: The Volumetrics Eating Plan: Techniques and Recipes for Feeling Full on Fewer Calories. New York, HarperCollins Publishers Inc., 2005, pp.8,16–17.*

55. Shick SM, Wing RR, Klem ML, McGuire MT, Hill JO & Seagle HM (1998). Persons successful at long-term weight loss and maintenance continue to consume a low calorie, low fat diet. *Journal of the American Dietetic Association*, 98, 408-413.

56. Simkin-Silverman LR, Wing RR, Boraz MA, Kuller, LH. Lifesyle intervention can prevent weight gain during menopause; results from a 5-year randomized clinical trial. Ann Behav Med 2003; Dec;26 (3): 212-20.

57. Sofi F, Cesari F, Abbate R, Gensini GF, Casini, A (2008): Adherence to Mediterranean diet and health statistics meta-analysis BMJ (Clinical research ed.) 337 (Sept 11: 2): a1344.

58. Tree nut consumption and weight management: A scientific review of the literatureby Michelle Wien, Dr.PH, RD,CDE & Joan Sabate, DrPH, MD appeared in Summer 2011.

59. U.S. Department of Health and Human Services and U.S. Department of Agriculture. Dietary Guidelines for Americans, 2005. 6th Edition, Washington, DC: U.S. Government Printing Office, January 2005.

60. Ulf Ekelund, et al. ,American Journal of Clinical Nutrition, April 2011 vol. 93 no.4, 826-835, Physical Activity and Weight Gain Prevention: Am Clinical Nutr 2011; 93(4) 826-835.

61. *Use of Nutritive and Nonnutritive sweeteners, Volume 104, Issue 2, Pages 255-275 (February 2004),* Journal of the Academy of Nutrition and Dietetics.

62. Vegetarian Science Daily (April 21, 2008) reports that Carnegie Mellon researchers Christopher L.Weber and H. Scott Matthews say that shifting from an American diet to a vegetable-based one would reduce greenhouse gas emissions equivalent to driving 8,000 miles per year.

63. Wahlstrom, Kyla L. & Begalle, M. (1999). More Than Test Scores – Results of the Universal School Breakfast Pilot in Minnesota. *Topics in Clinical Nutrition, vol* 15: no 1.

64. Weight Loss with a Low-Carbohydrate, Mediterranean , or Low-Fat Diet: New Engl J Med 2008; 359:229-241, July 2008.

65. What You Need to Know About Mercury in Fish and Shellfish, 2004 EPA and FDA Advice For: Women Who Might Become Pregnant, Women Who are Pregnant, Nursing Mothers, Young Children.

66. Wing RR & Hill JO. (2001). Successful weight loss maintenance. *Annual Review of Nutrition*, 21, 323-341.

67. Wyatt HR, Grunwald GK, Seagle HM, Klem ML, McGuire MT, Wing RR & Hill JO. (1999). Resting energy expenditure in reduced-obese subjects in the National Weight Control Registry. *American Journal of Clinical Nutrition*, 69, 1189-1193.

68. Wyatt HR, Grunwald OK, Mosca CL, Klem ML, Wing RR, Hill JO. (2002). Long-term weight loss and breakfast in subjects in the National Weight Control Registry. *Obesity Research*, 10, 78-82.

69. Wyatt HR, Phelan S, Wing RR, Hill JO. (2005). Lessons from patients who have successfully maintained weight loss. *Obesity Management*, 1, 56-61.

too Busy to Diet

A guide to smart nutrition when you're on the move.

Do you find yourself too busy to Diet? Are your days so packed with work, family, and social responsibilities that you grab unhealthy food choices in place of healthy meals?

The shift in how we live and work has made healthy eating and exercising a challenge. Too Busy to Diet is the result of the experience of two award winning nutritionist/diabetes educators with over 60 years of combined experience. it provides quick and easy solutions to the challenges we face in our busy lives.

it is written as a travel book for easy to access information that will help you navigate your day..

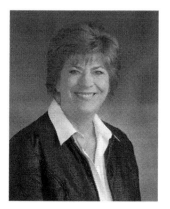

Jacqueline King is a registered dietitian, certified diabetes educator, and a fellow of the Academy of Nutrition and Dietetics. She has worked at Rush-Presbyterian St. Luke's Medical Center, Chicago, IL and Northwestern Memorial Hospital, Chicago, IL where she worked as the research dietitian at the Diabetes in Pregnancy Center.
She received her Bachelor's Degree in Medical Dietetics at University of Illinois at Chicago and her Master's Degree in Nutrition and Food Science at Northern Illinois University.

She has a busy nutrition consulting business in Glenview, IL. She sees private patients, consults to corporate health programs, and works with numerous businesses.

Visit her website at: www.Nutradynamics.com

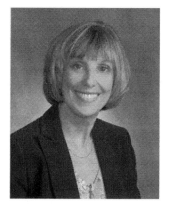

Monica Joyce is a registered dietitian and a certified diabetes educator. She received her Bachelor's Degree in Foods and Nutrition at Mundelein College/Loyola University in Chicago, Il. She received her Master's Degree in Human Services Administration at Spertus College in Chicago.

She is the Program Director of an American Diabetes Association Recognized Diabetes Program in an endocrinology practice in Chicago. She is a local and national speaker to health care professionals on diabetes. In 2004 she founded the Moses E. Cheeks Slam Dunk for Diabetes Basketball Camp for kids with diabetes.

Made in the USA
Lexington, KY
13 July 2014